The Transorbital Intracranial Penetrating Injury

This book is dedicated to my wife, children and four grandsons

The Transorbital Intracranial Penetrating Injury

A review of the literature from a neurosurgical viewpoint

By:

Martin Th. A. van Duinen MD PhD

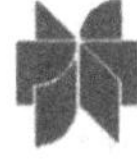

SPRINGER SCIENCE+BUSINESS MEDIA, B.V.

A C.I.P. Catalogue record for this book is available from the Library of Congress

ISBN 978-0-7923-5915-9 ISBN 978-94-011-4457-5 (eBook)
DOI 10.1007/978-94-011-4457-5

Table of contents

1. Introduction 1
2. Historical aspects regarding transorbital intracranial penetrating injury (TIPI) 7
3. Defining the concept of TIPI 12
4. Experimental research on cadavers 15
5. The nature of the penetrating object 20
6. Incidence 23
7. Anatomical data 27
8. Pathogenesis 39
9. Clinical presentation and initial evaluation 48
10. Physical examination 51
11. Neuroimaging 57
12. Treatment 71
13. Antibiotic therapy 78
14. Complications 80
15. Aggression 91
16. Accident 94
17. Fall injuries 96
18. TIPI caused by umbrellas 103
19. TIPI caused by pencils, slate pencils and ballpoint pens 105
20. Suicide by TIPI 108
21. Mortality and morbidity 113
22. Medicolegal aspects; prevention of TIPI 116
23. Brief review of a patient series from the literature 118

List of patients 124

References 138
List of reprints of illustrations from other authors 155
Index 159

1 Introduction

The brain, as befitting the most important organ of the human body, is well protected by a roughly spherical, thick, bony covering, consisting of the crown and the base of the skull, which shields against penetrating injury.

However, this strong, bony cover has several weak points at the cranio-facial transition, i.e. both orbits and the lamina cribrosa lying between them, which are areas of poor resistance. It is easy for a pointed, long, thin and strong object to penetrate into the brain via the orbit through the thin roof or the thin medial orbit wall via the paranasal sinuses. Penetration is also possible through the natural openings at the back of the orbit, i.e. the superior orbital fissure (SOF) and the canalis opticus (CO).

This is particularly true of children, whose immature orbits permit easy access to the intracranial cavity (Figure 1).

A penetrating injury of the orbit, thus, not only threatens the visual organ but can also be life threatening – in a case of perforation through the orbital wall – due to cerebral complications. Such an injury falls within an area of

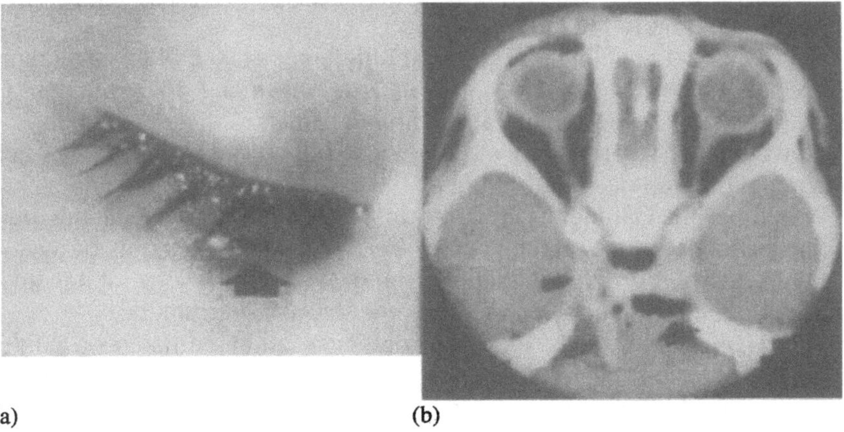

(a) (b)

Figure 1 Small lower eyelid wound, but deep intracranial penetration with the stem of a fern. (a) Photograph of right eye showing the site of penetration of the right lower eyelid (*arrowhead*). (b) Axial CT scan of the head, revealing a blood tract passing from the orbital apex through the middle cranial fossa into the posterior cranial fossa (*small arrowhead*). There is associated intracranial air (*large arrowhead*), but no evidence of a retained forreign body

overlap between the spheres of expertise of the ophthalmologist and the neurosurgeon and thus the patient should be examined and treated by both disciplines.

For the neurosurgeon, it is important to realize the high likelihood of infection associated with penetration through the orbit [1–3] and accompanied with, at least for war wounds, a mortality rate twice as high as that due to penetrating trauma through the crown of the skull (12.5% versus 6.4%) [4].

An ophthalmologist [5] is usually the first doctor to examine these patients, along with the family physician, pediatrician or emergency physician.

Often the patients initially present with an innocent-appearing wound involving the eyelid, though hiding a complicated, comminutive, impacted fracture of the orbit, accompanied by a severe brain lesion not yet manifest.

These doctors run a serious risk if they just treat the eyelid wound without considering a potential deep penetration. When this is suspected, a neurosurgeon should be called in for a consultation.

The ophthalmologist should remain involved in the care to prevent further damage to the visual organs and to promote healing of the orbital wound [5].

Detailed studies of penetrating orbitocranial injuries are scarce in the literature. Even the major textbooks rarely mention this type of trauma, with the exception of articles for example by De Villiers [2] and Chapman and Grove [6].

In Chapter 23, several smaller reviews of TIPI are cited, including Morrant Baker [7], Duke-Elder [8], Greig [9], Kjer [10] and Wesley *et al.* [11]. It is indeed a rare injury [12, 13].

Courville and Schillinger [14] found only one instance of an intracranial complication associated with an orbital lesion among 30 000 autopsies, and this was not even a perforating injury [12].

Rowbotham [15] reported only two patients with a transorbital injury among 1000 craniocerebral injuries.

McClure and Gardner [16] wrote in 1949: "Relatively little has been written about wounds which involve the intracranial structures by way of the orbits. This is difficult to understand since this is one of the most accessible modes of entry to the brain for stabbing instruments".

Kjer [10] noted in 1954 that: "No particular attention has been paid to this type of lesion; in the ophthalmologic and neurosurgical literature the contributions to the discussion are usually confined to case reports".

Lavergne [17] in 1959 stated: "Les traumatismes directs de la base du crâne avec l'orbite comme voie d'accès de l'agent perforant sont extrêmement rares".

De Villiers said in [2] 1975: "The literature on this subject consists mainly of individual case reports, few series comprising more than five cases have been reported".

On the other hand, however, he also remarks that transorbital stab wounds of the head as a group are extensively described in the literature.

AUTHOR'S NOTE

I can confirm the rarity of this lesion. During my 35-year career as a neurosurgeon, I never saw a single case. In contrast, Bard and Jarrett [12] treated 7 cases in 11 months and Bullock *et al.* [18] 5 cases in 5 years. Out of curiosity for this rather neglected subject in neurosurgery, I started an exhaustive literature search in order to add to the description of these injuries, thus filling a hiatus in the neurosurgical literature. The initiating impulse was given by press reports in the Netherlands about a possible accident (or attempted murder?) in which the autopsy revealed an intracranially positioned ballpoint pen having entered through the orbit.

The literature perused was primarily obtained as photocopies requested from the Royal Library in The Hague, The Netherlands. References at the end of these articles were used to track down further articles. In addition, I requested a corresponding literature list from the Library of Congress, Washington DC, USA, which was compared with my own literature collection. Several additional publications were found by this method.

Two dissertations on this topic were discovered, Wertheim's (Figure 2) written in 1904 [19] and Coqueret's (Figure 3) in 1905 [20]. Photocopies of these were obtained from Giessen (Germany) and Paris (France), respectively. Via the Internet, the large medical database in Minnesota was repeatedly searched with various key words (Medline, US National Library of Medicine, NLM). The university library in Keio, Japan (staff@med.keio.ac.jp) was extremely helpful in sending me Japanese literature. I could not read the Japanese texts, but fortunately Japanese authors tend to include a detailed English summary, usually very informative. Several Italian, Polish, Russian, Japanese, Norwegian and Czech articles had to be left out because they did not have an English summary.

In the collected patient series, primarily only those with a transorbital intracranial penetrating injury were included. The ophthalmologic literature contains many reports of penetrating injury of the orbits without intracranial complications. These injuries do not fall within the neurosurgeon's sphere of expertise and thus are not included in our patient database.

This volume includes many data from a large number of other authors. As far as possible, reference has been made to the respective author, trying not to compromise the readability of this work.

The neurosurgical literature contains many articles on penetrating injury through the cranial vault, but transorbital brain injury is rarely mentioned and then often just as a case history. We are concerned here with as thorough a literature search as possible to produce a sound description

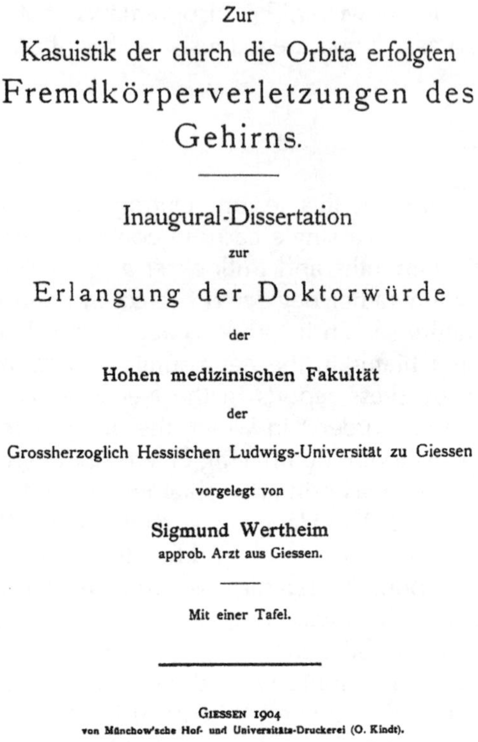

Zur
Kasuistik der durch die Orbita erfolgten
Fremdkörperverletzungen des
Gehirns.

Inaugural-Dissertation
zur
Erlangung der Doktorwürde
der
Hohen medizinischen Fakultät
der
Grossherzoglich Hessischen Ludwigs-Universität zu Giessen
vorgelegt von
Sigmund Wertheim
approb. Arzt aus Giessen.

Mit einer Tafel.

GIESSEN 1904
von Münchow'sche Hof- und Universitäts-Druckerei (O. Kindt).

Figure 2 Front page of Wertheim's dissertation

summarizing the clinical syndrome: the transorbital intracranial penetrating injury (TIPI). We shall also try to create a subcategory of fall traumata of children because of some of its characteristic features.

In Dutch literature, Verbiest [21] summarized the subject in issue. Two cases were reported by de Grood [22, 23] while Copper [24] presented a review of four cases in 1957.

To produce this study, more than 500 publications were examined (Figure 4). Of these, more then 160 were rejected once it became obvious that they did not contain specific information on the subject. The remaining 340 (360 at the end of the project) publications described 347 patients (Figure 5), constituting the basis of this investigation.

Near the end of the project, eleven new cases were added [23, 25–32]. The investigation being closed, details of these cases could only be partially assimilated into the present series.

The data of these 347 patients were handled in two ways. The general non-clinical data (author, year of publication, nature of penetrating object, right–left localization, type of trauma, etc.) were entered in tabular format in Microsoft Word 97 and processed with the sorting tool. A patient database

FACULTÉ DE MÉDECINE DE PARIS

Année 1905 THESE N°

POUR LE

DOCTORAT EN MÉDECINE

Présentée et soutenue le jeudi 14 décembre 1905, à 1 heure

Par MAXIME-PAUL COQUERET

Né à Caen (Calvados), le 24 octobre 1879
Ancien externe des hôpitaux de Paris et de la Maternité de l'hôpital Boucicaut
Médaille d'honneur des épidémies
Médaille de bronze de l'Assistance publique.

CONTRIBUTION A L'ÉTUDE

DES

PLAIES PÉNÉTRANTES DU CRANE

PAR LA VOIE ORBITAIRE

Président : M. LE DENTU, *professeur.*
Juges : MM. GUYON, BROUARDEL, *professeurs.*
ACHARD, *agrégé.*

PARIS
STEINHEIL, ÉDITEUR
2 RUE CASIMIR-DELAVIGNE, 2

1905

Figure 3 Front page of Coqueret's thesis

• Collected: >500 publications
• Not relevant: >160
• Included: 360

Figure 4 Literature

was concurrently established with Microsoft Access. For each of the 347 patients, as many clinical details as possible were recorded and processed with the queries tool of Access. The bar diagrams were prepared with Microsoft PowerPoint 3.

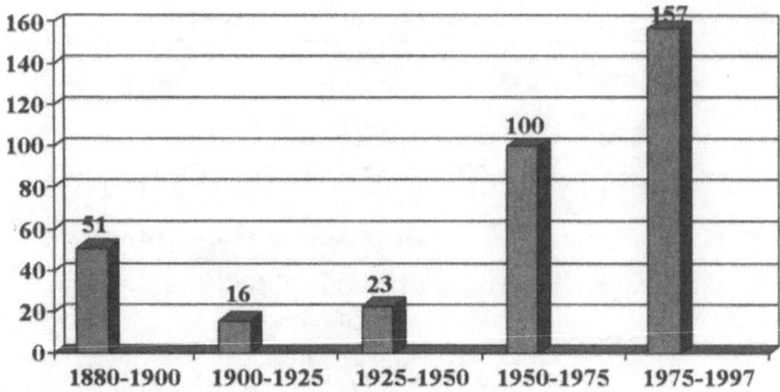

Figure 5 Year of publication; 347 patients

ACKNOWLEDGEMENTS

Special thanks go to the governing board of the Dr Eduard Hoelen Foundation in Wassenaar, The Netherlands. In a large measure, a donation from this Foundation helped the publication of this work. I owe grateful thanks and am in particular debt to J. A. M. Ceha MD, who critically reviewed the entire manuscript and annotated it in detail. Finally, without the excellent and greatly appreciated work of Mrs Alison Fisher, there would not have been an English translation.

Several illustrations were copied from publications by others. As much as possible, permissions to reprint were collected from authors and editors. At the back of this book, a table shows the exact origin of these figures. I apologize for the possible inferior quality of these reprints.

PERSONAL DATA

The author was trained from 1958 to 1967 in neurology, psychiatry and finally neurosurgery (supervisor: Dr A. C. de Vet, Senior Neurosurgeon) in the former St. Ursula Clinic, Wassenaar, The Netherlands; then practiced there as a neurosurgeon, becoming Head of the Neurosurgery Department in 1970. He obtained his Doctor's degree in 1976; thesis: The ependymoma of the cauda equina; promotor: Prof Dr H. Verbiest. In 1979, the Neurosurgery Department was transferred to The Hague, where the author remained Head of Department until his retirement in 1995.

E-mail address: mvduinen@wxs.nl

2

Historical aspects regarding transorbital intracranial penetrating injury (TIPI)

The history of this injury extends at least as far back as the story of David and Goliath in the Bible, 1 Samuel 17, verse 49. In that tale, David fells Goliath with a stone from a slingshot, hitting him on the forehead, causing the 2.78-m giant ("6 cubits and one span") to fall to the ground. The circumstances as pictured in the famous Dutch children's Bible by W. G. van der Hulst (Figure 6), however, cannot be correct. A stone thrown with that velocity could hardly have penetrated Goliath's thick frontal bone, let alone injured one or both frontal lobes. Even with a stone into a frontal lobe, Goliath would not have fallen down immediately. In addition, according to 1 Samuel 17, verse 5, Goliath waş wearing a copper helmet, which most likely also covered his forehead.

It is more probable, therefore, that the stone entered Goliath's eye socket and penetrated into the brainstem. For this to happen, David, being much shorter than Goliath, would most likely have stood on an elevation to give the stone a more horizontal and somewhat medially directed trajectory, in the direction of the brainstem. That David was actually standing higher than Goliath agrees with the description in 1 Samuel 17, verse 3. The text states that the Philistines and the Israelites both stood on mountain slopes with a valley between them. As Goliath approached the Israelites, then, he was standing below them.

In 1834, Scott [33] described two cases of TIPI. In his commentary he reports that Monro, Morgagni, Portal and Paré had already indicated the danger associated with an orbitocranial lesion, which could arise easily because of the "extreme thinness and delicacy of the bones of the face at this point". According to him, Webfer wrote in his "Observationes de affectibus capitis" that the Romans used to kill cattle for slaughtering by sticking a knife through the orbit into the brain.

Scott reported that in *De Sedibus et Causis Morborum* (1761), Morgagni cited in his 51st epistle many cases from earlier authors, but added that mostly the descriptions were inadequate. In the 57th section, Morgagni describes two cases. A pointed object in the eye socket injured one man. The eye was undamaged, but there was a perforation through the orbital roof. No symptoms were present for 3 days. On the fourth day the patient died. At autopsy, the diagnosis was meningitis, and a penetrating brain injury was found extending almost as far as the left lateral ventricle. Another

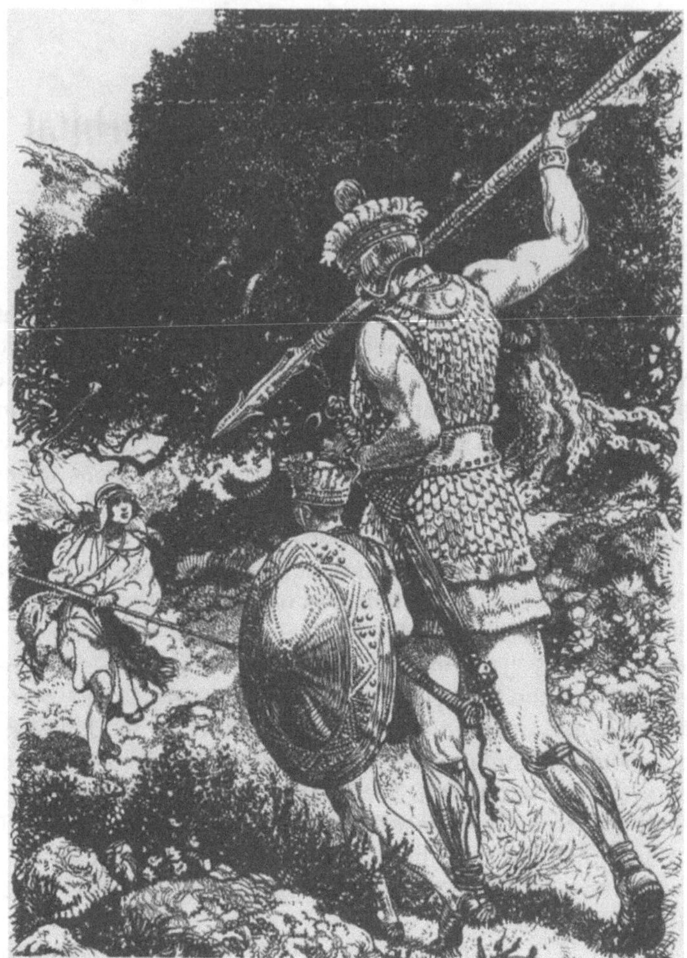

Figure 6 David and Goliath

man was stabbed with the point of a sharp sword through the left eye socket. He became comatose immediately, and died 10 h later. Autopsy revealed a brain lesion with intraventricular hemorrhage. These brief descriptions from Morgagni concisely stress the dangers of TIPI.

The famous case of the death of Henry II (June 30, 1559) of France is excellently described by Faria [34]. The probable manner of dying predicted by Nostradamus for Henry II was realized during a joust. According to Faria, his opponent's lance pierced through the king's helmet into the right eye. Coqueret [20 obs. 39) claims, however, that the outer corner of the left eye socket was injured. Scott [33], citing Paré, also states that the broken lance hit Henry II in the left eye. In Figure 5 from Faria's article [34],

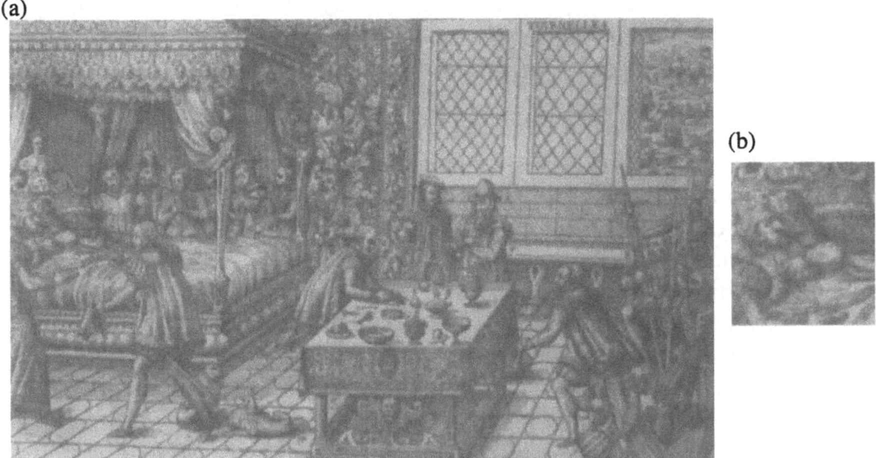

Figure 7 (a) The deathbed of Henry II; (b) detail

an ancient engraving from 1560 (Figure 7a); it would seem that Henry II's left eye was involved while the right eye appears to be intact. The autopsy report of Vesalius, who was called in for consultation, gives the left eye socket as the entry point, although the right orbit had splinters as well.

Paré and Vesalius could not save the king, although three prisoners were beheaded for experimental research. Henry II died 11 days later, probably because of meningitis and/or subdural empyema.

Morrant Baker [7] wrote in 1888: "Ever since men have fought and fenced, it has been known that the orbits present easy access to the brain". He describes 13 cases extensively (see Chapter 23).

Apprehension for a deep penetrating transorbital lesion can be found in the early literature. For example, Betke described in 1869 [35] a case involving a child who fell on the spout of an oilcan and he warned the mother: "Die Mutter wurde auf die Möglichkeit einer schweren Verletzung aufmerksam gemacht." (The mother was informed of a potentially serious injury.)

In 1897, an editorial appeared in *The Lancet* [36] containing a summary of TIPI, and giving the most essential features along with 8 case histories. In an earlier issue of *The Lancet* (July 1886), the danger of a penetrating orbital lesion had already been emphasized. It was stressed that small external orbital wounds can harbour a concurrent deep perforating injury. Perforation is likely because of the extremely thin bone of the orbital walls. In 1891, the associated mortality rate was over 90%, and in the course of more than ten years (1886–1897), no improvement had been made in the treatment. The author of the editorial ascribed this to a policy of wait and see and non-intervention. He pleaded for a more aggressive approach with inspection of the wound, removal of the foreign body and drainage. "Waiting for symptoms cannot be too strongly condemned in the light of our present knowledge." The prognosis could be improved by surgical intervention.

In 1897, Winkfield cited Hulke [37], who produced the following pithy summary: "In no class of cases is the surgeon more likely to be put off his guard. At first all that may be apparent is a slight injury to the external parts – a trifling wound of the upper lid, and sometimes not even this, for the instrument may have slipped under the lid and left merely a patch of ecchymosis in the conjunctiva. Brain symptoms may be absent. Two or 3 days may pass over, during which the patient goes about as usual. Then brain symptoms make their appearance, sometimes suddenly, and the patient dies in the course of a few hours or days and the true nature of the cause is revealed only in the postmortem room."

In 1904 Wertheim's thesis [19] appeared. He exhaustively described a case of perforating orbital injury, in which the patient fell in a bush and a branch entered the temporal lobe through the superior orbital fissure (SOF). He added descriptions of 11 cases from the literature, of which 5 could be traced in our search [38–42].

Coqueret's thesis, *Contribution à l'étude des plaies pénétrantes du crane par la voie orbitaire* [20], written in 1905, deserves detailed mention. For the first time, an extensive and recapitulating study was written about all aspects of TIPI based on 79 cases, which were mostly collected from the literature up to that time. Meningitis and abscess formation were considered the greatest threat, but quick intervention could improve the prognosis. Penetration generally occurred through the orbital roof or the medial orbital wall, through which the anterior cranial fossa can be reached. Penetration was said to occur rarely through the SOF or optical canal, with injury in the temporal fossa. Most often the orbital roof was penetrated as the object frequently came from below, combined with the "mouvement de recul instinctif" (instinctive reaction of recoiling) with the head thrown back. There is always an eyelid injury (except with bullet wounds) because of a second reflex: the instinctive closing of the eyes when an object approaches.

Of the 79 cases, 16 patients had suffered a bullet wound, and thus they will not be included in this study. In the remaining 63 patients the injuries were caused by umbrella ($n=13$), pitchfork ($n=6$), spear ($n=3$), sword ($n=7$), pipestem ($n=4$), iron rod ($n=3$), wooden object ($n=5$), bayonet ($n=4$), pen ($n=3$), other objects ($n=15$). Thus, the umbrella is obviously a dangerous object.

Coqueret cites Berlin (*Verletzungen der Orbita*, 1880) who ascribed 49% of injuries to aggression and 45% to falls.[1] Coqueret found that 44%

[1] Graefe u. Saemisch, Handbuch der ges. Augenheilkunde Bd 6, p. 630, 1880. Berlin's original text was unavailable to us.

involved cases of aggression, 67% accidents and 30% falls. In these percentages, patients are obviously counted more than once and bullet wounds are included, which we shall not consider here.

The external wound is often slight, heals quickly and usually fades in time, becoming invisible even under a magnifying glass. The orbital roof or the medial orbital wall shows a comminuted fracture with pieces of bone pushed inwards. Usually the frontal lobe is pierced, especially when an umbrella is the agent of injury, as it generally penetrates the orbital roof. It is also possible that the ventricle system is reached. The eyeball is often spared, but not vision, due to a direct optical nerve lesion. Coqueret exhaustively treats the consequences and the complications, which he classifies into early (infectious and non-infectious, such as paralysis and carotis cavernous fistula) and late (brain abscess, epilepsy).

According to Berlin (cited by Coqueret), the prognosis of 62 orbital roof perforations was poor: 41 patients (66%) died. [Note: Dietz [43] states that Berlin treated 52 patients with more than 80% mortality, including 83% brain abscesses and 11 cases of meningitis. Thus, 20% of the patient group survived, but half of these were invalids. However, these included other injuries as well as transorbital perforations.]

Coqueret [20] reported a mortality of over 82%, three quarters of whom died of 'meningitis–encephalitis'.

He paid a great deal of attention to the treatment of TIPI. Of 85 cases of cranial injury in his time, only 5 patients underwent trepanation. In 1888 Quénu was already arguing against the trend towards non-intervention for general penetrating skull injury; according to him, prompt trepanation and drainage led to better results. Coqueret wondered whether this also applied to TIPI. He could not answer this question due to a lack of data, but 3 of the 5 surgically treated patients recovered satisfactorily, which he found encouraging. He recommended immediate operation in order to take care of the orbital–cerebral injury and drain the anterior cranial fossa. This requires a frontal trepanation, which was carried out in those days with hammer and chisel.

This operative technique was first described by Polaillon, among others, in 1891 [20 obs. 10, 44] but actually performed by his colleague, M. Poirier. The latter operated on a patient stabbed by an umbrella, by applying a large frontal skin flap and performing with a hammer and chisel a trepanation "of the size of a five franc silver coin". He then opened the dura and removed impressed fragments of bone and damaged brain tissue, tied up a bleeding artery and inserted a drain. One day later a drain was also inserted into the orbit. The patient healed successfully.

This was one of the first reports of this technique being applied for TIPI, along with Laplace's description [45] in 1891 of a temporal trepanation for a case of TIPI. Winkfield [37] applied a similar technique in 1897. These are also some of the earliest descriptions of trepanation in general. I do not know whether these authors were aware of Wagner's 'pioneering osteoplastic craniotomy', which was published several years earlier in 1889 [46].

3

Defining the concept of TIPI

Let us begin with a precise circumscription of what we understand here by the concept: transorbital intracranial penetrating injury.

This study concentrates on TIPI caused by objects whose diameter is smaller – often much smaller – than the diameter of the anterior orbital opening (about 35–40 mm) and which thus, in principle, leave the orbital rim intact. We are exclusively dealing with civilian injuries, usually involving thin, long, strong, most likely pointed objects travelling at low velocity, that traverse the orbit and end up intracranially.

Stab wounds involving blunt objects or knifes with a broad blade differ considerably from stab wounds involving pointed thin slim objects that penetrate the orbit with minimal force [47]. Blunt objects require more force to penetrate the orbit and produce a wound with a larger diameter than the object itself, possibly with damage to the eyeball, eyelid avulsions, etc., causing more intracranial damage.

Duke-Elder [8] classified low-velocity penetrating injuries as puncture wounds, divided into *stab* wounds with sharp pointed objects and *lacerated* wounds with blunt objects. Generally, the penetrating object has a low velocity and the head is stationary, but the opposite is also possible. The head can be impaled on a stationary object; this is termed an impalement injury [48] or Phälungsverletzung [43, 49]. A typical example is a child falling on a pencil. In the literature, high-velocity injury (HVI) has been called a penetrating injury [50], and low-velocity injury (LVI) a perforating injury, but, in this study, we shall make no distinction between 'penetrating' and 'perforating'. The term transorbital intracranial penetrating (perforating) injury (TIPI) is the best description of the injury in question. The label 'transorbital intracranial injury' is incorrect as it embraces more possibilities, including injuries caused by an object whose diameter is larger than the anterior orbital opening, which are not considered in this study. The term 'penetrating' was added here to emphasize that we are concerned only with penetrating objects whose diameter is smaller than the orbit's entrance.

Consequently, this study will not address to the following injuries:

1. Penetrating orbital injury limited to the orbit. Such a lesion is a purely ophthalmologic matter and is not handled in neurosurgery. In 1924, Greig [9] divided penetrating orbital injuries into traversing and non-traversing types. The latter affects the structures of the orbit but is not life threatening. In his view a traversing injury is defined as having

breached the dura (or passed the boundary of the superior orbital fissure or the optic canal), penetrating intracranially and then must be considered as an open skull wound.

2. Extensive blunt facio-orbital injury involving fractures elsewhere in the face along with a transorbital lesion.
3. Extensive blunt orbital lesion caused by objects whose diameter is greater than the orbit, seriously damaging the orbit through compression, with possible intracranial penetration.
4. High-velocity injury (HVI) to the orbital region. An HVI produces quite different and more serious damage remote from the path of the projectile, due to the effect of shock waves and temporary cavitation produced by radial forces in a cylindrical zone around the missile's path. Strain develops, resulting in damage to the surrounding tissue with a concentric zone of coagulation necrosis. In contrast, in a low-velocity injury (LVI), the damage is restricted to the path of the penetrating object [51–53] as a local zone of hemorrhagic necrosis [51, 54]. Thus, the prognosis after LVI is in principle more favourable than after HVI. With HVI, the eyeball is often penetrated, while in LVI the eyeball is more likely to be displaced, although often leading to serious damage to the retrobulbar neural and vascular structures.

   The amount of kinetic energy delivered by the penetrating missile equals ½ × mass × velocity^2. Thus, velocity makes the greatest contribution to the kinetic energy [5, 52]. The kinetic energy can be high (military weapons, hunting rifles), average (handguns) or low. Here, we shall deal only with the last category.

   It is difficult to make a clear cut-off between LVI and HVI.

An impact velocity of more than 100 m/s, especially more than 320 m/s, is necessary to produce an explosive type of lesion with shock waves and tissue cavitation, producing concentric necrosis [55]. Arrows fired with a modern compound bow have an average discharge velocity of 60–90 m/s [55] and thus a lower impact velocity. Injuries caused by arrows have therefore been included in this study, although the discharge velocity is close to the limit of 100 m/s and thus could cause some damage of the kinetic type [61].

TIPI caused by air rifle pellets is not considered here.

In the literature a few cases are reported in which a foreign body first penetrates the sinus maxillaris or nasal cavity and, after traversing the orbit, ends intracranially. These cases are included in this study.

It might be questioned whether low-velocity TIPI is actually a separate entity or not. However, many authors treat TIPI as a separate nosological category [10, 16, 56] due to the following characteristics:

1. The special anatomical relationships;

2. The nature of the trauma, i.e. low-velocity stab wounds;
3. The insidious initial course with few symptoms;
4. The discrepancy between the apparently slight external wound and the severe cerebral complications that can arise later;
5. The frequently appearing complications that – certainly in earlier times – led to high mortality;
6. The high chance of liability issues.

These factors indeed are aspects of TIPI which are totally different from the usual penetrating injury of the crown of the skull.

Several quotations from the literature support the opinion that TIPI forms a special, separate clinical picture:

Verbiest [21]: "Transorbital stab wounds make up a separate section."

Matson [57]: "Special note is made of the importance of small penetrating injuries which may occur in childhood as the result of falls on small sharp objects."

De Villiers [2}: "Transorbital stab wounds deserve to be regarded as a special category due to the frequent occurrence of complications and the high mortality caused by them."

Gouazé and Santini [58]: "Les traumatismes orbito-encephaliques constituent une entité qui doit être isolée."

Duke-Elder [8]: treats TIPI in a separate chapter.

Bullock *et al.* [18]: "Transorbital intracranial injury, produced by low velocity objects, presents a unique clinical problem."

Scarfo *et al.* [50]: "A special nosolopical category."

Unger and Umbach [59]: "Eine Sonderstellung nehmen Fremdkörper ein, die den Orbitabereich hirnwärts überschritten haben."

Dietz [43]: "Die orbito-frontalen perforierenden Verletzungen stellen eine Sonderform der fronto-basalen Schädelhirnverletzungen dar."

Michon and Liu [60]: "Orbitocranial foreign bodies constitute a special class of injury that requires careful attention."

4
Experimental research on cadavers

As early as 1877, Annandale [41] casually described tests made on a 'dead body' in which he stuck a knitting needle through the middle part of the upper eyelid into the brain. According to him, the needle tended – if it was not pushed with force – to slide along the orbital roof and to penetrate through the SOF (superior orbital fissure) or OC (optic canal).

In 1879, Steavenson [61] reported his experiments followed by examining the brains of cadavers. He too inserted a knitting needle through the orbit. Left to follow its own course when being pushed through the orbit, the needle always entered intracranially by the wide medial side of the SOF, passing under the brain parallel with the n. oculomotorius, reaching the medulla oblongata.

Only when the needle was forced in a certain direction could it pass through the lateral part of the SOF, penetrating through the sylvian fissure and injuring the Broca region and striate body. It is hard to understand why he required a hammer to perforate the orbital roof. Greig [9] indicated as early as 1924 that this did not agree with 'clinical evidence of injuries received *in vivo*'. It is possible that Steavenson was experimenting on cadavers fixed in a certain manner with formaline, which could make the tissue particularly hard.

In 1895, De Nobele [62] experimented with metal rods on a cadaver. He described how easy it was – to his surprise – to reach the SOF. If the rod was inserted somewhat diagonally from below through the medial part of the lower eyelid, an identical lesion was always created, as appeared in his case 2: through the basal medial side of the brain it penetrated as far as the occipital bone, 15.5 cm deep. Sometimes the path deviated somewhat because of the bony structures of the sella or the os petrosum.

In 1900, Martial [63] described his detailed experiments. He confirmed that effort was required to penetrate the orbital roof of cadavers with a 'pointed instrument', but added this was caused by the formalinization procedure. The formalinization applied in those days also produced artifacts in the brain tissue. If the instrument (injection needle or a metal rod) was not inserted close to the medial canthus and pushed in an almost sagittally, slightly oblique upwards direction, the SOF and CO were not reached and penetration did not take place. Also trying to proceed along the orbital roof was not successful with these formalinized cadavers due to the great resistance of the tissues.

By varying the course slightly, the intracranial path could be altered. Martial listed the following results:

A. Experiments 1 and 2: the 'coupe du pédoncule' (Figure 8). A rod was inserted through the medial right and left canthus to a depth of 15.5 cm, as measured from the lower edge of the orbit. The following occurred:
   1. Tearing of the chiasma
   2. Possible injury to the mammillary body
   3. Piercing of the homolateral peduncle
   4. The homolateral occipital lobe could be damaged in the second temporo-occipital convolution under the splenium.

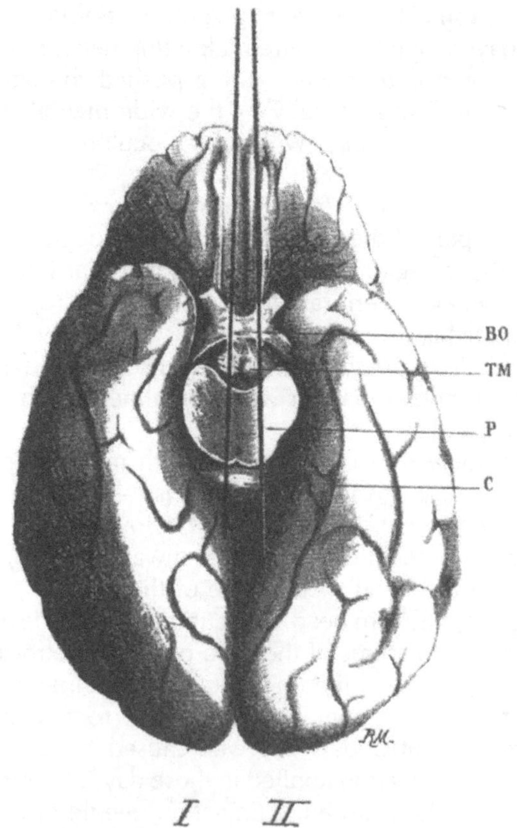

Fig. 1 et 2. — Face inférieure du cerveau — les tiges sont figurées par un trait noir — la coupe du pédoncule a été pratiquée là où les tiges ont passé.
BO, Chiasma et bandelettes optiques. — TM, Tubercules mamillaires. — P, Pédoncule. — C, Corps calleux.

Figure 8 Martial's coupe du pédoncule

B. Experiment 3: A rod was inserted through the medial canthus 14 cm deep along the orbital floor. The path was:
   1. The basal part of the temporal lobe
   2. Caudate nucleus
   3. Lateral ventricle, posterior horn and regio calcarina. A stab with a fencing foil could follow this path.

C. Experiment 4: Penetration to a depth of about 14 cm via the lateral lower orbital rim, from outside to inside. The chiasma and optical tract remained intact, but the peduncle was pierced and the cerebellum was penetrated.

D. Experiment 5: A rod was inserted to 15 cm depth, from inside to outside, and to some extent from underneath upwards. The following occurred:
   1. Penetration of the foremost part of the sylvian fissure
   2. Proceeding under the second temporal convolution intracerebrally
   3. Then through the first temporal convolution extracerebrally
   4. Finally, the object came to rest in the second occipital convolution.

   Martial states aphasia could be the clinical result of these injuries.

E. In the following experiment, the rod was inserted 15 cm through the medial part of the orbital floor from below upwards and from inside to the midline into the contralateral hemishere, producing the following pathway:
   1. Penetration of the innermost 'corne sphenoidale'
   2. Damage to the optical tract and the central grey matter
   3. Through the contralateral mammillary tubercle and the internal capsule
   4. Through the contralateral peduncle
   5. Into the cerebellum.

F. Penetration via the sylvian fissure was also possible, resulting in damage to the basal ganglia and the internal capsule, through the lateral ventricles and terminating approximately in the cuneus.

In summary, Martial proposes that the following structures are practically always affected:

1. Chiasma or the tractus opticus
2. Peduncle
3. 'Corne sphenoidale'
4. Internal capsule
5. Thalamus
6. Corpus striatum.

In addition, the cavernous sinus and the internal carotid artery can be punctured. Martial anticipates that the mobility and elasticity of the artery might occasionally save it from injury (Figure 9).

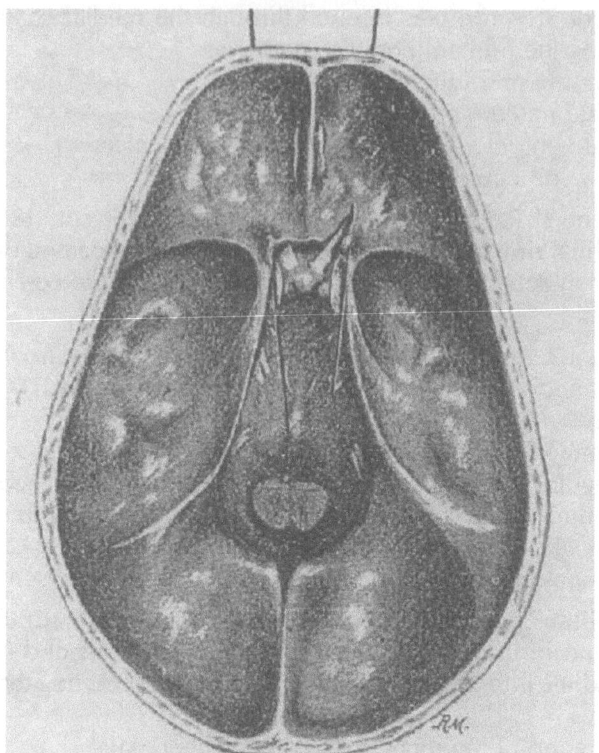

Figure 9 Puncture of the sinus cavernosus

Greig [9] summarized Martial's experiments in English in his article, but since then Martial's work has not been cited.

Solieri [64] distinguished three zones at the base of the skull through which intracranial penetration can occur: a frontal facial, a middle jugular and a posterior occipital zone. The facial zone is the most dangerous one and the easiest to penetrate because of the presence of the orbits, sinuses and the cribriform lamina. Solieri [64] also experimented with transorbital brain injury (1914); he carried out tests on cadavers with a pitchfork prong.

1. A horizontal direction from front to back through the left bulbus produced the following: the object passed through the SOF, lateral from the internal carotid artery in the sylvian fissure along the middle cerebral artery, without damaging it. Through the anterior part of the second temporo-occipital convolution and the innermost part of the nucleus amygdaloïdeus, the optical tract was reached and the peduncle was perforated. Finally, the object stopped in the occipital lobe.

2. An oblique direction upwards and inwards into the right orbit: the object penetrated through the orbital roof 1.5 cm in front of the optic foramen

and entered the first frontal convolution, crossing the midline to enter the contralateral hemisphere after injuring the third frontal convolution, ending in the oval center.

3. An oblique path upwards and outwards in the left orbit. Through the SOF, the penetrating object can reach the temporal fossa and temporal lobe.
4. Via the upper inner rim of the right orbit. The object reached the cavernous sinus through the optic foramen, and the internal carotid artery was injured. Subsequently, the penetrating object passed over the edge of the petrosal bone in the posterior cranial fossa through the peduncle and the cerebellum.
5. Along the lower border of the right orbit, the pitchfork prong passed through the ethmoid bone along the clivus and ended in the pons.

Stab wounds through the orbit thus produce very deep-seated brain injury at a variety of locations, depending on the direction of and the depth reached by the penetrating object. It follows that the clinical neurological symptoms are very variable and are not easily classified into one system [64].

Nakayama *et al.* [65] remarked that, practically speaking, any intracranial area can be reached through the orbit, depending on the length and the direction of the penetrating object.

5

The nature of the penetrating object

In the literature a wide range of objects is presented, as shown in the following random list:

Paint brush [45], point of an ornamental star from a car fender [66], rose bush branch [67], bakelite door handle fragment [68], ferrule end of fishing rod [37], afrocomb [69], wire rod [70], tip of pool cue [71], glass rod [72], knife [e.g. 73], umbrella ribs and ferrules, metal rods [74, 75], wire [12], theatre sword [76], golf tee [77], pitchfork [10], arrow [55, 75], metal fragment, chisel [78], screwdriver [71], pencil, slate pencil, ball point pen, table fork, chopstick [79, 80], scissors [71], tree branch [71] bamboo stem [81], foil, glass fragment [59 case 5, 82], nail [83], knitting needle, straw [84], pipe stem [e.g. 85], car antenna, teaspoon [86], broken ruler [84], piece of ice [87], ski pole [88], welding rod [88], gear stick [88], bicycle pump rod [49], billiard cue [71], kangaroo tooth [89], wooden toy [90], brake handle of bicycle [91], grass stubble [16 case 2], plastic handle of lights lever [92], spout of oil can [35, 93], iron spike [78], steering wheel lock [94], merchandise display hook [95], crochet hook [96], upturned clothes dryer [97], metal motorbike stand [98], handle of water faucet [99], sled runner [12], red hot iron nailrod [100], coat hook [78], ice pick [56], walking stick [101], tent pole spike [102], toothbrush (Figure 10) [103], harpoon [104, 105], top of a soft-drink bottle [106], garden cane [107], fern [25], door key [26], oven door spring [108], needlefish [29].

A TIPI with a CCF, caused by a very remarkable penetrating object (sharp beak of a needlefish) was published by McCabe [29]. A ten-year-old boy was struck by a needlefish in the right eye, causing immediate loss of consciousness and a homolateral flaccid paralysis. Angiography showed a left-sided CCF plus evidence of cerebral infarction. The boy died after 10 days. Autopsy revealed an injury of the right orbit, crossing the midline through the sinus sphenoidalis, causing injury to the left hemisphere and creating a CCF in transit.

Another curious transorbital penetrating object was a kangaroo tooth, published by Lawson [89]. A driver of a motor vehicle collided with a kangaroo. A tooth fragment from the kangaroo traversed the orbit and probably through the SOF; it became lodged intracranially in the pole of the temporal lobe.

Wooden objects will be treated separately as wood is a particularly dangerous material. Thus, it is important to know the nature of the penetrat-

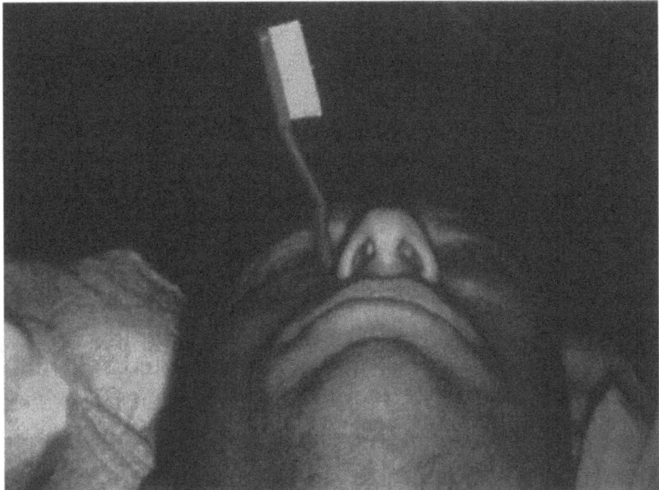

Figure 10 TIPI with a toothbrush

ing object. Because of its porous, organic structure, wood harbours many microbes (aerobic and anaerobic) and fungi, thus encouraging infection after perforation. Wood is generally soft, fragmenting and splintering easily under light pressure, but it can also be simply formed into a pointed end. The splintering makes it difficult to remove all of the bits. A wooden object in the orbit can be bent by the wall or perforate it and/or partially splinter. The organic material will naturally produce a greater tissue reaction than an inorganic foreign body. According to Miller *et al.* [108], wood is associated with a greater morbidity than other materials, just because of the infections it causes.

Wertheim [19] found, in his patient series, that 44% of the penetrating objects were made of wood. In our series, this proportion was 35%. Tracing and removing the wooden penetrating object are thus important tasks. However, wood is difficult to locate radiologically and thus presents difficulties for neuroimaging. Radiologists should be aware of the problems that can arise when tracing a wooden foreign object and the risk of misinterpretation when evaluating the scan images.

In De Villiers' [2] patient series – 10 patients with a transorbital injury – the penetrating object was a knife in seven cases.

Birch-Hirschfeld [110] noted the following distribution among 172 orbital stab wounds, (which, however, also include non-traversing injuries):

Umbrella	28	Knitting needle	10
Thrust weapon	27	Wood splinter	10
Pitchfork	24	Pencil	7
Iron rod	17	Nail	6
Knife	10		

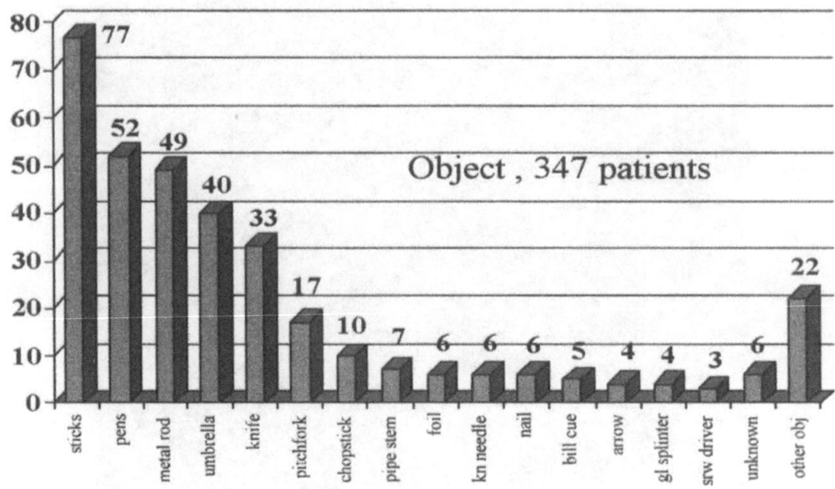

Figure 11 The nature of the penetrating object

Our patient series, 347 cases, showed the following distribution (Figure 11):

Stick	77	Knitting needle	6
Pencil	52	Foil	6
Metal rod	49	Billiard cue	5
Umbrella	40	Arrow	4
Knife	33	Glass splinter	4
Pitchfork	17	Screwdriver	3
Chopstick	10	Unknown	6
Pipestem	7	Other objects	22
Nail	6		

6
Incidence

Gouazé and Santini [58] state that "La pénétration de corps étranger dans la boîte cranienne par l'orbite est relativement frequente" (TIPI is relatively frequent) and De Nobele [62] agrees, but practically all other authors working with TIPI point out the rarity of this injury, e.g. Dujovny *et al.* [13]: "Intracranial penetration of a foreign body via the orbit is a rather unusual event during time of peace".

Approximately 2% of all patients attending an Emergency Department suffer from a penetrating injury somewhere on their body [111]. Penetrating injury of the abdomen and thorax (35.6%) is 4 times as common as a cranial penetrating injury (8.6%) [111]. From Tomita and Miwa's data [112 Table 3] it can be deduced that 35% of all cranial penetrations pass through the orbit. However, De Villiers reports 10.7% [2] and du Trevou and van Dellen 19% [48].

Due to its rarity, it is difficult to estimate the incidence of TIPI. In addition, a number of TIPIs go unrecognized, being without cerebral symptoms. Sometimes it is evident from the length of a deeply located and barely protruding removed object that intracranial penetration must have occurred [113: an object of 6 cm].

As another example, Wertheim [19] cites a case of Lawson, in which an 8.5-cm-long wooden pen of 1 cm diameter was removed from the orbit; the patient, however, showed no cerebral symptoms.

Agarwal *et al.* [114, case 1: a 7-cm-long foreign body], Johnson [cited in 19] and Sedan and Paillas [115] have also reported these types of cases. Sedan described a case where a 6-cm piece of pipestem was removed from the eye socket of a 26-year-old woman without cerebral symptoms. J. B. Marin initially reported this case in 1713.

Several authors affirm that it is primarily children who suffer TIPI [2, 6, 116, 117]. Of all eye injuries, 66% occur in patients 16 years old and younger, with a peak incidence between 9 and 11 years [90]. Eye injuries occur 3–4 times more often in men than in women, but this difference disappears in the age group 6–8 years [118]. Among children, 10% of all eye injuries are caused by branches, sticks, pencils, etc. [118]. It is difficult to estimate the percentage of orbitally penetrating injuries that lead to intracranial damage [116].

Examining the age distribution of the current patient series (only 315 of the 347 patients, as age was not always noted) (Figure 12), it is apparent

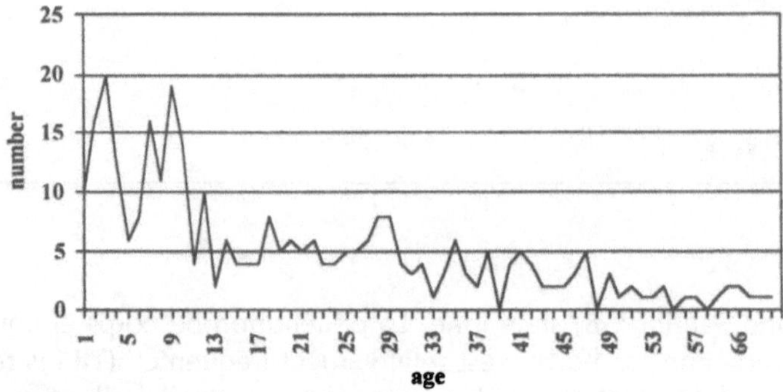

Figure 12 Age of TIPI cases; 315 patients

that the risk of TIPI is greatest for children between 1 and 13 years old, with a peak from 3 to 9 years. However, the total number of patients younger than 16 years old equals the total number of those between 16 and 79 years old. Thus, the treating physician has an equal chance of encountering a patient presenting with TIPI in either age category.

GENDER

The occurrence of TIPI is 4 times more frequent for males as compared with females (Figure 13).

DISTRIBUTION BETWEEN THE RIGHT AND LEFT ORBITA

In our series, the right orbit was involved more often than the left. In subsequent chapters it will become clear that considerable differences in the right–left preference arise from the various causes of TIPI (Figure 14).

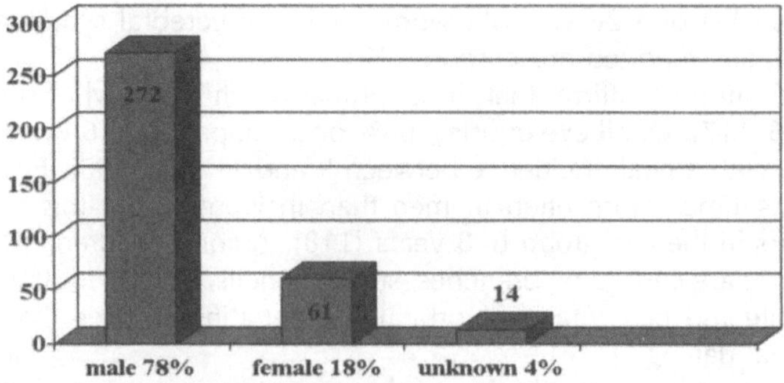

Figure 13 Male/female distribution; 347 patients

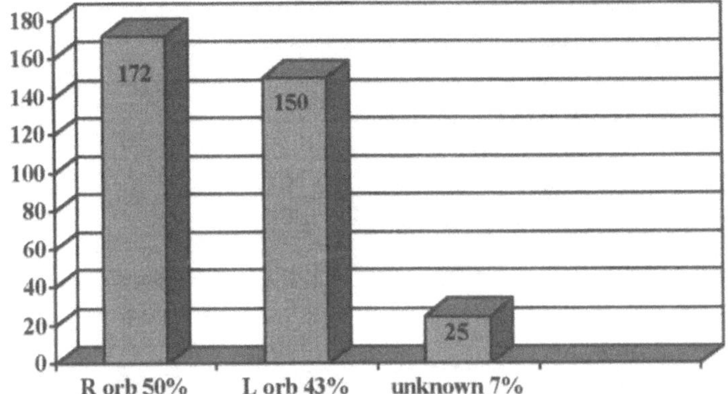

Figure 14 Right/left orbita distribution; 347 cases

THE AGE AND GENDER DISTRIBUTION OF 246 PATIENTS FROM THE TOTAL POPULATION PRESENTING WITH TIPI

In the age group 6–8 years, there is a difference between boys and girls, in contrast to previously described findings in cases of injuries limited to the eye [118] (Figure 15).

Four groups of TIPI can be distinguished, according to the cause of the injury (Figure 16):

- Fall trauma
- Accident (industrial, traffic, home, freak accidents)
- Criminal aggression, altercation
- (Attempted) suicide.

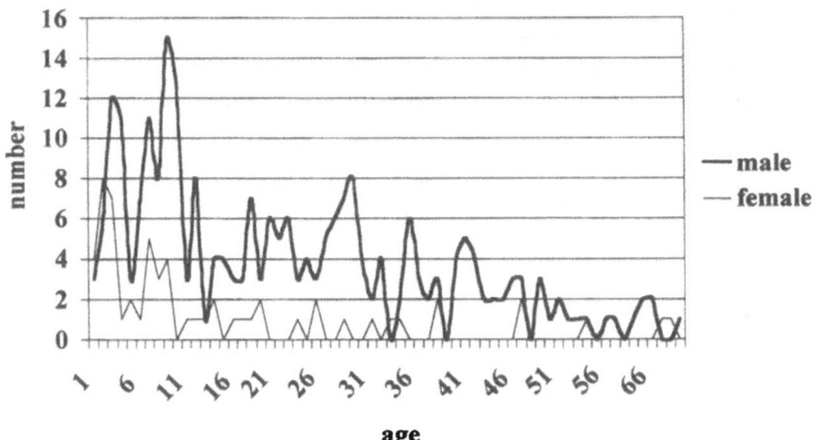

Figure 15 Age and gender; 246 male, 59 female, 42 unknown age and/or gender

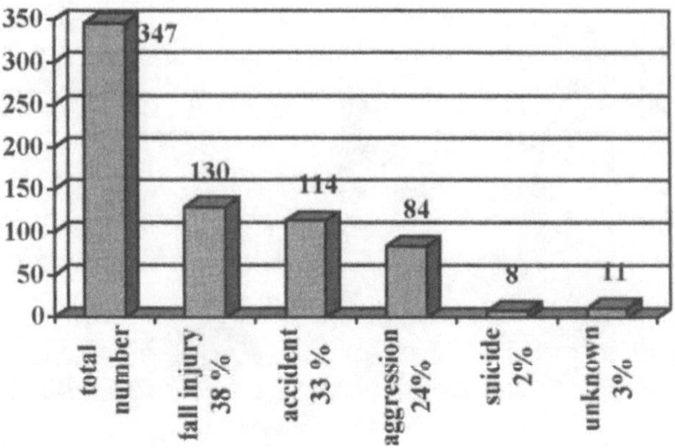

Figure 16 Four groups of causes of TIPI

Table 1 Causes of TIPI

	Present series (%)	De Nobele (Berlin) (%)	Coqueret (%)	Sollman (%)
Fall trauma	38	45	30	
Accident	33		67	
Aggression	24	50	44	33
(Attempted) suicide	2			

In the present series, fall trauma was the cause in 130 patients (38%), accident in 114 patients (33%), aggression in 84 patients (24%) and suicide in 8 patients (2%).

In the literature, other percentages can be found.

De Nobele [62] cites Berlin who recorded, for 69 cases, 50% aggression and 45% accident and fall trauma.

Coqueret [20] noted in his series 30% fall trauma, 44% aggression and 67% accident as etiologies; in these percentages, patients are counted more than once.

Sollman *et al.* [119] reported aggression as responsible for 33%. However, these values from the literature are based on smaller series than the present one (Table 1).

7
Anatomical data

In this chapter, we treat anatomical details relevant to the understanding of the transorbital intracranial injuries. Both orbits and the lamina cribrosa between them form an area of minimal resistance in the cerebrum's bony protection, through which a penetrating agent can easily reach parts of the brain situated behind and above the orbits. The orbit's anatomy has a significant effect on the development of a transorbital brain injury, so let us review several salient features of importance for the neurosurgeon. We shall not go into an exhaustive description of the orbit's anatomy. This can be found for example in Winckler [120] and Lagrange [121].

The eye socket is generally described as a horizontal rectangular pyramid (it is more triangular at the back) situated behind the protruding orbital rim with a posterior–medial axis. The anterior cranial fossa and the frontal sinus bound the orbit on the upper side, the temporal fossa at the rear and the ethmoid sinus medially. The apex terminates at the sphenoid sinus and the floor of the eye socket is the roof of the maxillary sinus (Figure 17).

The eye socket, housing, nourishing and protecting the eye with the adnexa and the orbital fatty tissue, is formed by seven separate pieces of bone of the face and cranium. Some 50% of the bony wall of the orbit borders on brain tissue and its blood vessels [122]. In anthropoids the eye sockets lie more precerebrally, while in humans they are infra- and precerebral [124].

The shape of the orbits is often given as conical [121], funnel-shaped or pear-shaped, the stem of the pear being the optic canal [123]. The geometric apex of the orbit lies at the most medial and widest part of the superior orbital fissure (SOF) [121] and not at the canalis opticus [CO], an anatomical detail of great pathogenic significance in the transorbital intracranial penetrating injury.

Notably, this conical shape of the orbit will cause more or less sagittally penetrating objects to be funneled backwards [10] and medially towards the apex with its concentration of vessels and nerves, which can therefore be easily damaged [123]. In addition, the presence of an anatomical opening there, the SOF, allows the penetrating object to pass easily intracranially.

Strictly speaking, the orbit is neither a cone, because its width (38–40 mm) is greater than its height (33–35 mm), nor an exact pyramid. The geometrical pyramid form matches it best [124], however, and simplifies the description of the anatomy and the consequences of this specific trauma [121].

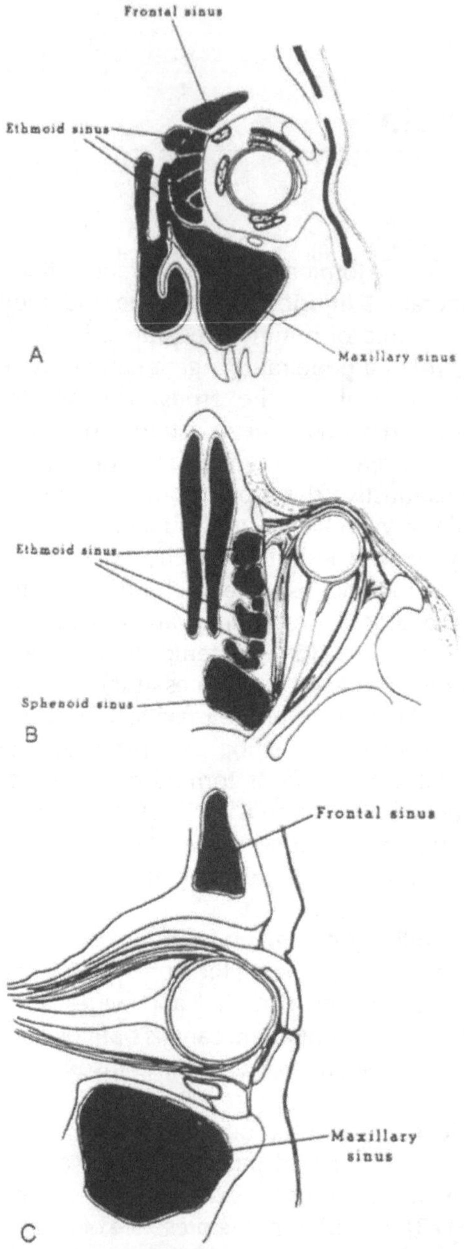

Figure 17 The structures surrounding the orbit. (a) Coronal section through the head demonstrating relationship of frontal, ethmoidal, and maxillary sinuses to the orbit. (b) Axial section showing relationship of ethmoidal and sphenoid sinuses to the medial wall of the orbit and the orbital apex. The optic canal indents the lateral wall and sphenoid sinus, and may traverse the medial wall of the last ethmoid air cell in 4 per cent of the population. (c) Sagittal section through the relationship of the frontal and maxillary sinuses to the orbit

Thus, four walls can be (artificially) distinguished in the eye socket, roundly blending from one into another, with the exception of the border between the floor and the lateral wall, which is perpendicular and where the inferior orbital fissure (IOF) is located. The medial wall runs approximately in the sagittal plane, while the lateral wall forms a 45° angle with the sagittal plane.

Seven bones make up the eye socket: os frontale, ala major and minor of the sphenoid bone, maxilla, os palatinum, os lacrimale, os zygomaticum and the ethmoid [125] (Figure 18). Together, they form the curved orbital walls with different radii towards the apex.

The orbital roof is triangular and dome-shaped, and is mostly formed by the orbital plate of the os frontale and at the back partly by ala minor of the sphenoid [120].

The floor of the orbit is primarily made up of the orbital plate of the os maxillare (infero–medial), the os zygomaticum (antero–lateral) and the

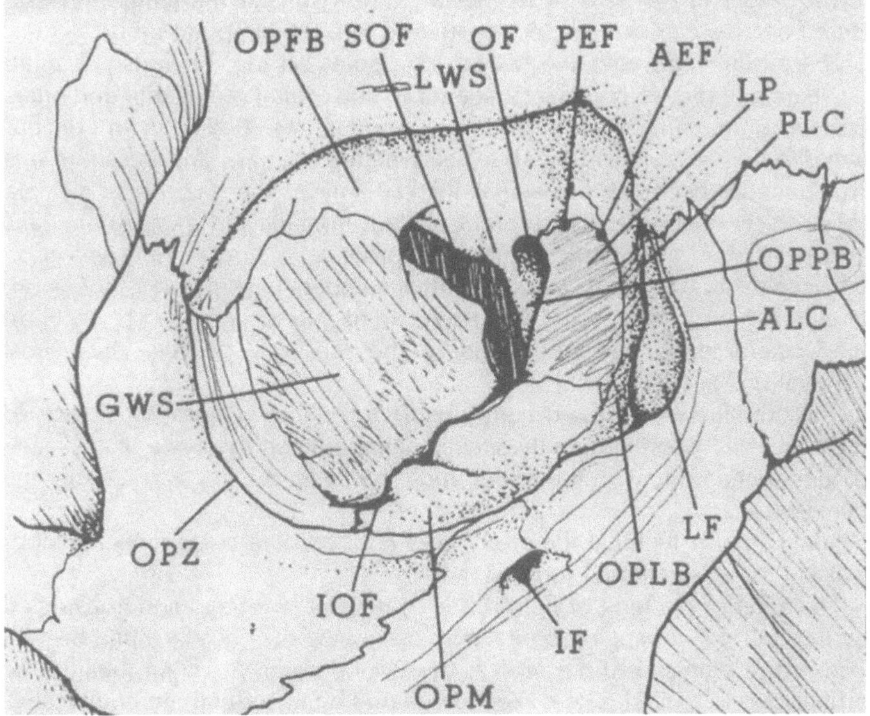

Figure 18 Schematic view of the bones of the orbit. LP = lamina papyracea; GWS = greater wing of the sphenoid; LWS = lesser wing of the sphenoid; OPZ = orbital plate of zygoma; OPFB = orbital plate of frontal bone; OPM = orbital plate of maxilla; OPLB = orbital process of lacrimal bone; OPPB = orbital process of palatine bone; OF = optical foramen; SOF = superior orbital fissure

os palatinum (posterior), bordering the sinus maxillaris. The floor is slightly concave in front and slightly convex at the rear [62]. It is the weakest part of the orbit, especially along the groove of n. infraorbitalis [126]. Blow-out fractures generally occur through the medial part of the orbital floor. Perforating injuries, on the other hand, will rarely go through the orbital floor, for reasons to be discussed later.

The medial wall consists mostly of the lamina papyracea of the ethmoid, forming the dividing wall to the ethmoidal bone cells (Figure 19). According to Coqueret [20], this bony wall is only 0.002–0.004 mm thick; but it is fortified by the buttressing effect of the ethmoidal air cells [125]. The very thin lamina cribrosa separates the ethmoidal cells from the intracranial space. An upwardly angled and medially penetrating object can thus easily pierce first the lamina papyracea and then the lamina cribrosa, crossing the midline to reach the brain. The lateral orbital wall is mostly made up of strong bony tissue (the frontal process of os zygomaticum, ala major and part of os frontale). However, the uppermost part of the rear, forming the lower border of the SOF, is thinner and approximates the temporal fossa. Here fractures can occur with penetration into the temporal fossa.

The orbital roof, with the frontal lobe poles on top, obviously is quite vulnerable and deserves special attention. The orbital roof is thin and offers little resistance against a penetrating force (Figures 20–22). With conventional radiographs, it is difficult to see whether fractures are present in this thin bone. It becomes somewhat thicker only at the back, near the ala minor. It can incorporate extensions of sinus frontalis and sinus ethmoidalis [12, 127]; thus perforating injury can produce a direct communication between the brain and the sinuses, with accompanying high risk of infection. In elderly people, the orbital roof even can disappear partially [11, 128]. In the posteromedial part, the bone of the roof is especially thin; most penetrations occur here [6].

The orbital roof is thus usually unable to deflect penetrating objects to the rear. Perforation frequently occurs, depending on the angle of approach of the foreign body with the orbital roof; the larger the angle, the easier the penetration.

Some authors feel that the orbital roof is so thin that it is practically nonexistent for a penetrating force [11].

The anterior opening of the orbit is somewhat protected and constricted by the strong overhanging orbital rim, narrowing the entry in some degree. The widest diameter of the orbit is thus found about 1–1.5 cm behind the orbital rim [121, 123]. The protection offered by the orbital rim could cause penetrating objects to angle off and enter through the eyelids or the conjunctiva [129]. The inferior orbital rim is the weakest section; when penetration occurs through the orbital rim, it is most likely to be here [130].

In children, the orbital roof is very thin and partially absent. In addition, the protecting supraciliary ridge is yet underdeveloped.

(a)

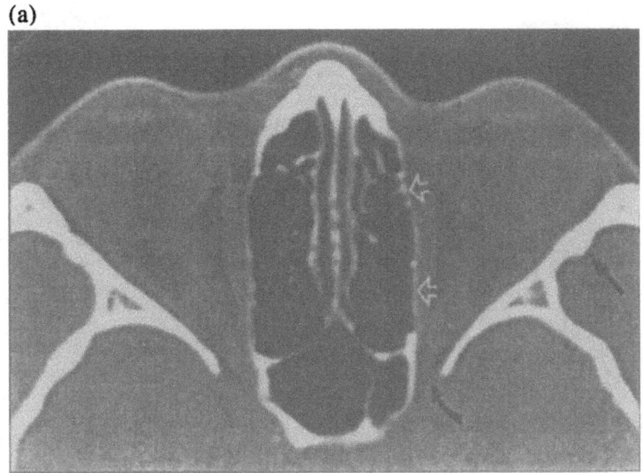

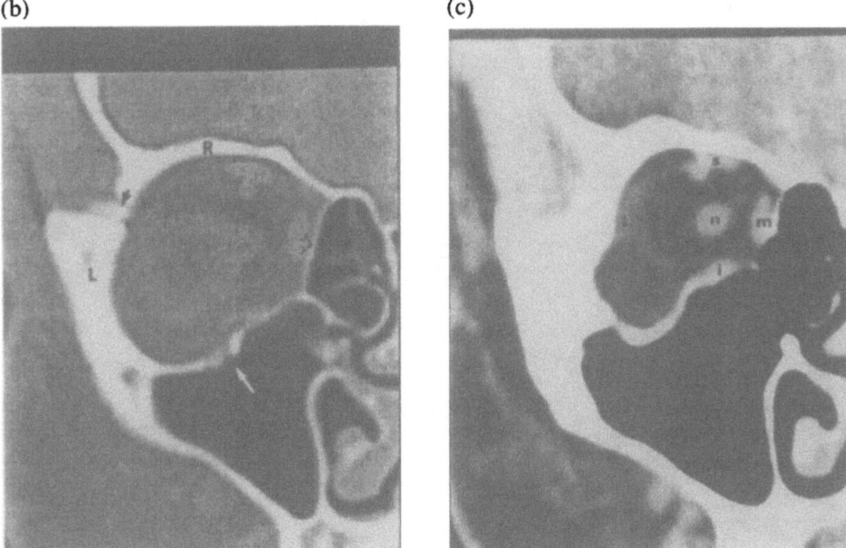

Figure 19 CT imaging of the normal anatomy of the orbit. (a) Axial CT, bone window settings, shows the thin medial wall (open arrows). The lateral orbital wall (straight black arrow) and the SOF are seen well. (b) Coronal CT (bone window settings) shows the thick lateral orbital wall (L) and roof (R). Note the thin floor with the grooves (white arrow) for the infraorbital nerve. The thin medial wall is seen well. (c) Coronal CT (soft tissue settings) shows medial (m), inferior (i), lateral (L) and superior (s) rectus muscles. The optic nerve (n) is seen well and surrounded by fat

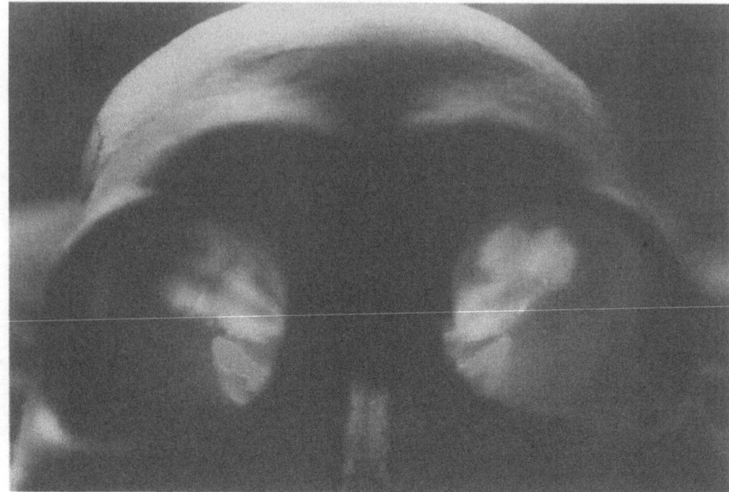

Figure 20 The orbital roof from outside

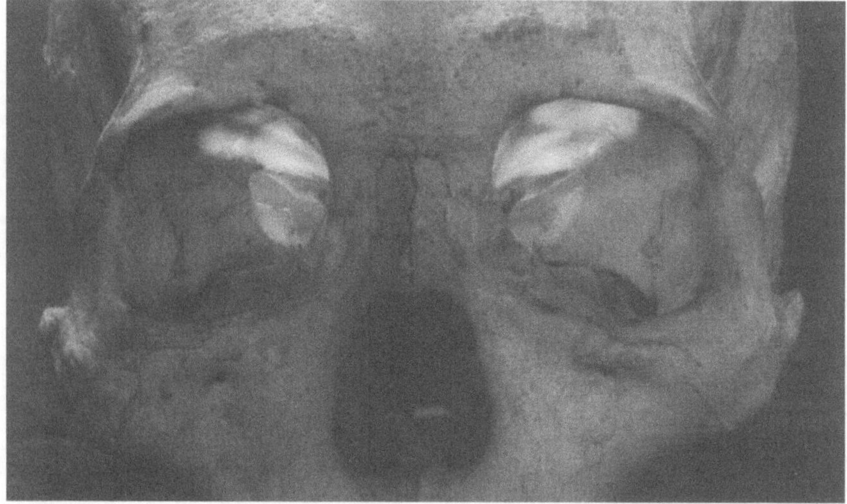

Figure 21 The orbital roof from outside

The dura lying upon the orbital roof is thin and adherent. It is especially thin medially on the lamina cribrosa because of penetrating filaments of n. olfactorius. Thus, in an orbital roof fracture, the dura is easily torn. It has a poor healing tendency, often worsened by interposition of arachnoid or brain tissue [11, 127].

In clinical practice, the thin structure of the orbital roof was used to advantage. In 1933, Dogliotti [131] applied the 'puntura transorbituria' for

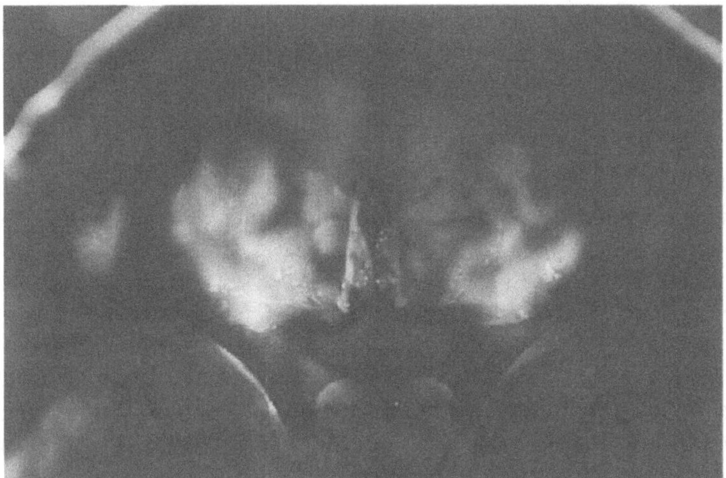

Figure 22 The orbital roof from inside

direct pneumo-ventriculography. He punctured the frontal horn of the lateral ventricle directly through the orbital roof (Figure 23a).

Fiamberti [132] adopted this technique for his transorbital prefrontal leucotomy in psychiatric patients (1937). The idea of treating psychiatric patients by frontal leucotomy originated with Moniz, but he carried it out

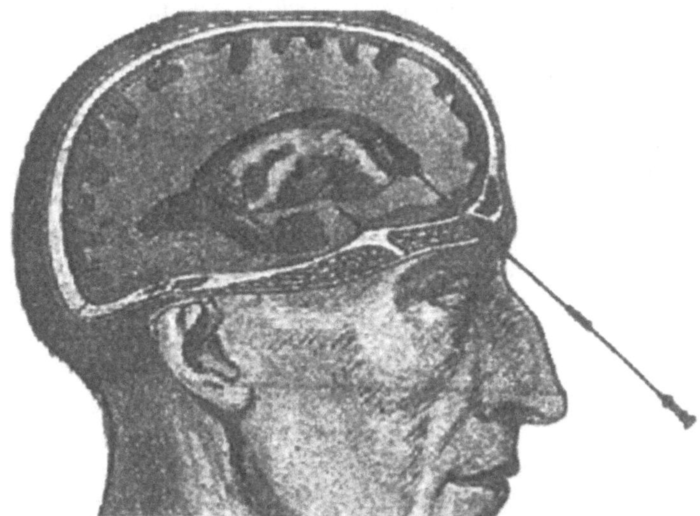

Figure 23a The 'puntura transorbituria' of Dogliotti

through a frontal trepanation. Freeman [133] utilized the transorbital leucotomy extensively, perforating the thin orbital roof. Complications were seldom reported.

In 1995 a new method was developed involving transorbital puncture via the SOF, in order to reach the sinus cavernosus for embolization treatment of a carotis cavernosus fistula [134].

In this neurosurgical study, the orbital contents require only limited description.

Its volume is about 35 cc [135], of which only 7 cc (20%) are taken by the eyeball. The remaining 28 cc contain muscles, nerves, fat, glands and blood vessels [135]. The orbit can thus accommodate a relatively large foreign body without showing great disturbance of function [136, 137].

The eyeball is a strong elastic ball situated in a pool of fatty tissue, with a characteristic structure: it is well lobulated and easy to displace [135]. A pathological process outside the muscle cone can produce shifting of the eyeball in the frontal plane; a space-occupying lesion inside the muscle cone causes a more axial proptosis. A pointed object entering the orbit at low speed is more likely to cause the eyeball to shift (to the side and/or the front) than to penetrate it, unless it is, for example, a knife with a broad blade [1, 2].

The distance from the eyeball to the medial orbital wall (6.5 mm) is slightly larger than the distance to the lateral wall (4.5 mm). Therefore, it is plausible that a medially penetrating object will injure the eyeball less frequently than an object entering laterally [103]. In our series, 5% of medial TIPIs were associated with damage to the eyeball, versus 6% with lateral TIPIs, not an impressive difference.

The vital orbital structures lie behind and medially from the eyeball. Thus, it could be surmised that a median sagittal penetrating injury is more likely than a lateral penetrating injury to damage the important retrobulbar orbital structures [47]. Our patient series did not support this hypothesis. Combined n2 and n3, n4 and n6 injuries indeed occurred three times as often with medial eye socket perforations compared with lateral penetrating injury. This, however, can be explained by the fact that, in general, medial eye socket perforations occurred three times more often.

The laterally entering TIPI even has a greater chance (48%) than a medial one (34%) of being associated with retro-ocular nerve damage.

The n2 is mobile in the orbit but is fixed at the foramen opticum and thus cannot avoid here external forces. Close to this posterior part of the n2 lies the first undivided section of the n3. Thus, a combined injury is likely to occur at this point.

At the back of the orbit, two anatomical openings present for potential penetration to the intracranial cavity, without bony fracture.

The superior orbital fissure (SOF) is the common access point.

Greig [9] indicated as early as 1925 the importance of the SOF in traversing orbital wounds. According to this author, the SOF allows a rod of 10 mm in diameter to pass without fracturing bony structures. In the skulls available to us for examination, the SOF diameter was at most 5 mm.

The SOF has a keyhole shape, is approximately 22 mm long [103], is widest on the medial side and is found superolaterally at the end of the eye socket. The fissure is limited by the inner edge of ala major and the lower edge of ala minor. The n3 and n6 along with the first branch of n5 pass through the medial part of the SOF. The n4 runs through the SOF more laterally and thus is somewhat better protected (Figure 23b). Several smaller vessels and nerves are not given in detail here (n. nasociliaris, v. ophthalmica, a. lacrimalis, etc.). Through the SOF runs an elongation of the dura mater from inside to outside.

A very important anatomical detail concerns the venous space of the sinus cavernosus, connected to the rear of the SOF on the inferomedial side [134, 138]. The arachnoidal space of the temporal fossa connects more laterally to the SOF. A medially penetrating object through the SOF would, therefore, perforate the sinus cavernosus and possibly the a. carotis. A more laterally penetrating agent would end in the temporal lobe or between the medial temporal lobe and the lateral wall of the sinus cavernosus (Figure 23c). The penetrating object can also pass extradurally through the SOF, making it invisible [139] but possibly still palpable during trepanation [12 case 6, 57, 72].

Looking at a skull into the orbit reveals that access to the SOF is maximally 'open' and thus easily penetrable by a more medially entering agent

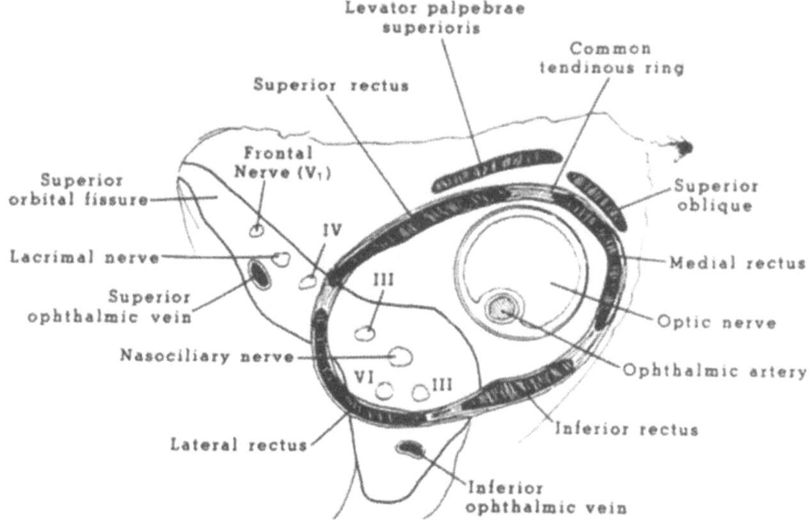

Figure 23b Position of the n. trochlearis in the superior orbital fissure

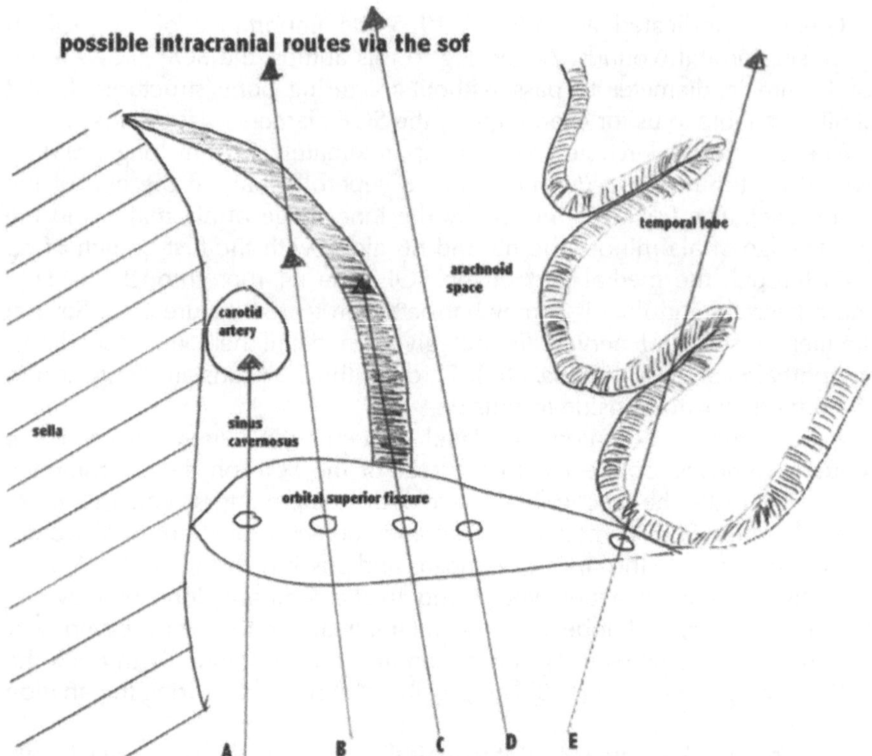

Figure 23c Intracranial routes via the fissura orbitalis superior. (a) Via the medial SOF in the sinus cavernosus with carotid artery injury. (b) Via the medial SOF in the sinus cavernosus with or without perforation of the sinus wall to the posterior fossa. (c) Localization of the foreign body in the dura of the sinus wall. (d) Perforation into the arachnoid space, eventually into posterior fossa. (e) Via the lateral part of the SOF in the temporal lobe

(Figure 24). For a laterally penetrating agent, access to the SOF is much smaller, although then the optic canal is maximally accessible (Figure 25). The consequences of this peculiarity for lateral or medial TIPI will be discussed later.

Martial [63] already indicated in 1900, in his cadaver studies, that the SOF is most easily penetrated via the medial canthus. The walls of the SOF are relative strong, thus occasionally the penetrating agent becomes stuck in it [19].

The canalis opticus (CO; Figure 25b) has relative strong walls and is rarely penetrated [140, 141], although there are some contradictory reports [116, 142]. Through the intact unfractured CO, the homolateral temporal lobe cannot be reached – due to the direction of the optic canal in the

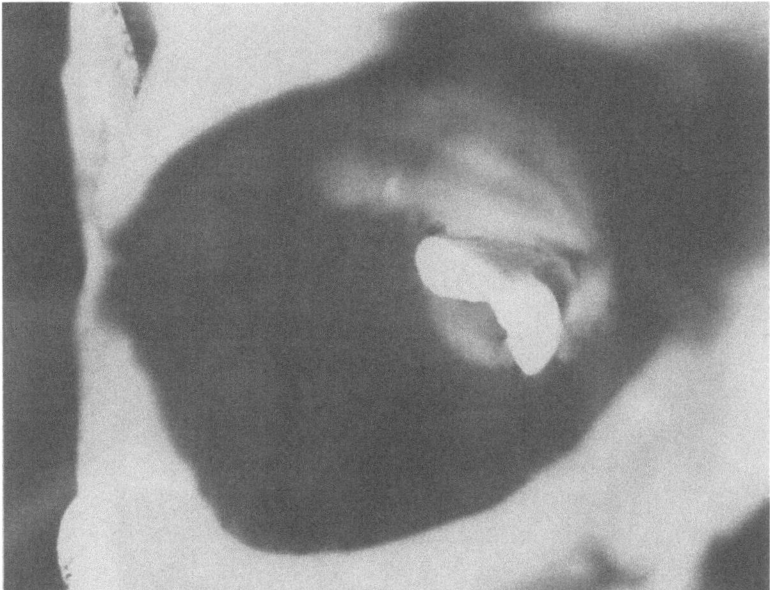

Figure 24 The superior orbital fissure, seen from the medial part of the anterior orbital opening

bone – even though some authors consider otherwise [143]; to be discussed later.

The inferior orbital fissure (IOF) has a very modest role to play in transorbital injury. Through this fissure the fossa pterygo-palatina [144] and the infratemporal fossa [125] can be reached.

The penetrating object must have a certain minimum length in order to traverse the orbit. It is therefore important to have an idea of the orbit's anteroposterior dimensions. Various authors have explored this theme.

- Merkel [cited in 62 and 19]: In men, the depth of the orbit is 43 mm, in women 40 mm.
- De Nobele [62]: The depth of the orbit varies in the literature from 39 mm (Emmert) to 50 mm (Richet, Tillaux). De Nobele himself found a distance of 45 mm, as measured from the innermost canthus to the CO. As measured from the outermost canthus, it is 49 mm. In children, objects of 25 mm in length can pass through the orbital roof [145]. In adults, the minimum length is 50 mm.
- Wolfe [124] reported that the depth of the orbit was never more than 46 mm.
- Simonton and Arthurs [123] noted that the distance from the lower orbital rim to the CO was approximately 50 mm.
- Lasky *et al.* [103]: "The average adult orbit is 40–45 mm in depth."

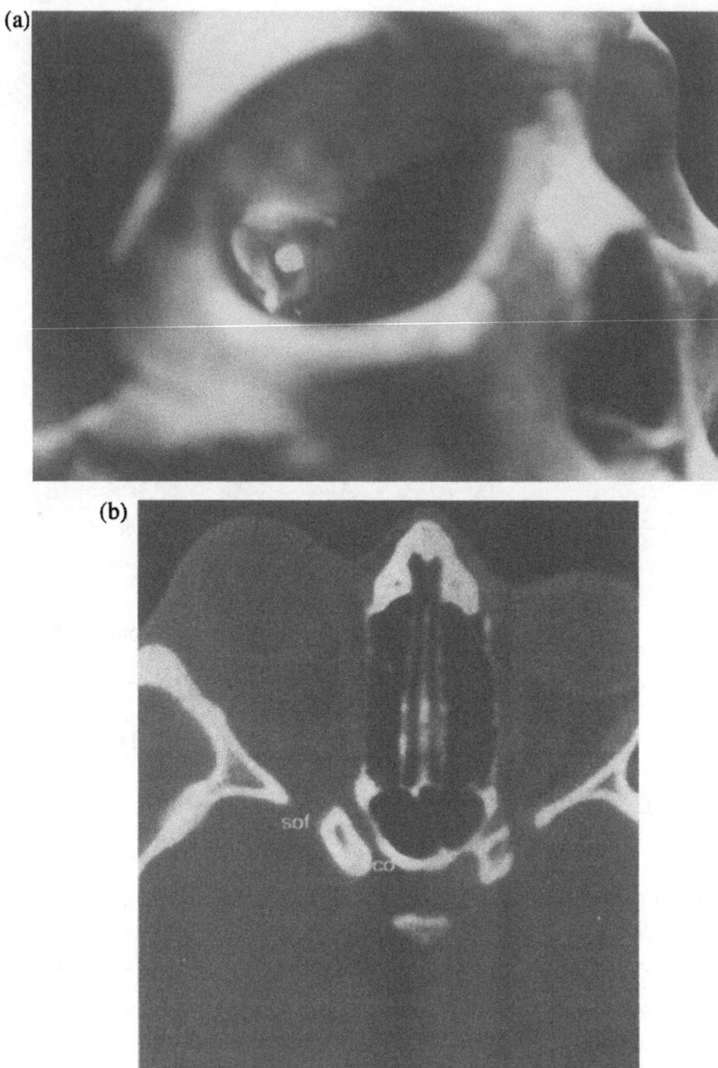

Figure 25 (a) The canalis opticus seen from the lateral orbital rim. (b) The optic strut, flanked by the superior orbital fissure and canalis opticus

– My own measurements of several skulls produced a result of 53–55 mm.

It is reasonable to assume that penetration has occurred for objects longer than 45–50 mm in adults; in children a shorter length is applicable.

8
Pathogenesis

Many authors have pointed out that the pyramidal structure of the orbit forces long and thin perforating objects towards the back and the apex [e.g. 1, 148], easily leading to damage of the ocular nerves n2, 3, 4 and 6 and extraocular muscles, and to subsequent intracranial penetration. A foreign body, entering sagittally, can obviously penetrate quite deeply, as can an obliquely entering object, by deflection off the converging orbital walls; depending on its angle, force, form, size and consistency.

A knitting needle, a fencing foil or a spoke can penetrate more deeply than a twig or a piece of wood, which breaks easily [110]. The eyeball can be easily pushed aside, but, on the other hand, by its position, form and the hard sclera it can also contribute in deflecting the penetrating object towards the orbital walls [99, 116, 146].

The walls of the pyramid, particularly the roof and the medial wall, are thin, and can be penetrated by a sturdy object entering with a certain amount of force at a reasonably large angle to the wall. A less-strong wooden object splinters easily, leading to multiple intra-orbital and/or intracranial fragments.

The sturdy sloping (45° to the sagittal plane) lateral wall, primarily formed by ala major, is not easily perforated; here an approaching object is likely to be deflected towards the widest medial part of the SOF, where intracranial penetration can then occur easily. The lateral wall may also be responsible for the tendency of objects to slide along it, to cross the midline after intracranial penetration through the SOF and injure the hypothalamus, with all its associated serious consequences [2].

Penetration sometimes occurs through the orbital rim, followed by secondary penetration into the orbit [130], especially at its weakest point, the lower section. In adults, the other three orbital rim sections are generally strong enough to deflect approaching objects, leading to penetration of the upper or lower eyelid [129] or, as is the case with children, equally through the edge of the orbit [147].

Cases of infraorbital penetration, i.e. from the outside through the orbital floor, passing transorbitally and ending intracranially, have been described [148].

Occasionally, a knife thrust through the outer side of the lateral orbital rim will traverse the homolateral orbital contents and pass through the contralateral orbit, finally ending in the lower frontal part of the contralateral hemisphere [149].

There is no consensus in the literature regarding the most frequent point of entrance for penetration of the anterior opening of the orbit. According to De Nobele [62] and Martial [63], penetration usually occurs through the medial canthus after deflection of penetrating objects by the strong base of the nose and the sturdy orbital rim. These structures form a sort of trap net or pit with a sturdy rim and an easily perforated weak floor, leading to medial canthus perforation.

De Nobele [62] is of the opinion that the small apophyses of the os frontale and os zygomaticum, forming the lateral orbital rim, deflect objects readily towards the temporal fossa, which could explain the low frequency of laterally penetrating injuries of the orbit.

Duke-Elder [137] also agreed that larger objects generally penetrate through the inner canthus; according to him penetration through the upper or lower eyelid is much less common, while penetration through the lateral canthus is rare.

Würdemann, as cited by Colley [150], claimed that, in 75% of affected patients, penetration occurred through the medial upper eyelid.

Hoffman *et al.* [47] stated: "A higher percentage of penetrating injuries to the medial upper lid, as compared with injuries to the lateral upper or lower lid, result in either orbital injury or intracranial injury."

Dimitrakopoulos *et al.* [136] maintained that foreign bodies usually penetrate via 'the lower region of the orbit', and less often via the medial wall or the orbital roof. Superolateral penetration would be rare due to the protection offered by the strong orbital wall there.

Other ophthalmologic authors [52, 151] report that "penetrating orbital injuries of the upper eyelids have a greater tendency to intracranial extension than those of the lower eyelids." However, due to the blink reflex, covering most of the anterior opening of the orbit with the upper eyelid, *a priori* the number of perforations through the upper eyelid will be greater and consequently a greater number of intracranial perforations will be seen. No information is available as to the percentage of intracranial penetration for equal numbers of upper and lower eyelid perforations.

Unger and Umbach [59] stated that a perforating injury of the lower eyelid is often associated with an intracranial injury via the SOF.

Dietz [43] was of the opinion that the 'typical' state of affairs is for a foreign body to penetrate through the medial upper eyelid from lateral–low to medially upwards and to the rear.

Mutlukan *et al.* [152] presented the (in his view) first case of penetration through the lower eyelid, with preservation of the eyeball and perforation of the orbital roof. In our patient series, this was noted 13 times, including in earlier literature.

Sarda *et al.* [113] held that perforation generally occurs through the lower outer region of the orbit or through the inner canthus, and rarely through the upper–inner region of the orbit, because of its protection by the orbital margins. He described a case, in which penetration occurred at an (according to him) unusual site, i.e. the upper and inner quadrant of the orbit, perforating the upper lid. This is, however, in our series, the most frequent course.

The eyelid closure reflex is clearly faster than any low-speed object, thus resulting in many upper eyelid lesions. De Nobele [62] stated that, in 75% of cases, the upper eyelid was perforated. The blink reflex covers the eye with a rather strong layer of skin thus providing some protection against a penetrating force.

Sometimes the eyelids are not injured, however, and penetration occurs through the conjunctiva or the fornix. In these cases, any deeper penetration may go unnoticed.

In our series, 284 patients suffered penetration through the anterior opening of the orbit. (Note: incomplete descriptions and other forms of penetration among the 347 cases were not included.)

Perforation occurred through the:

Upper eyelid in 45% (median : lateral = 3 : 1)
Lower eyelid in 21% (median : lateral = 3 : 1)
Conjunctiva in 17% (median : lateral = 5 : 1)
Both upper and lower eyelids in 11%
Uncertain in 6%

In this series, medial penetration occurred 4 times more frequently than middle and lateral perforation. We conclude that, indeed, the medial upper eyelid is penetrated most often in TIPI.

The orbital wall can be penetrated at various locations. In our patient series, the following distribution found in 296 of 347 patients is shown in Table 2.

Table 2 Location of penetration of orbital wall

	No. cases	Percentage
Orbital roof	149	50
SOF	89	30
Med. orbital wall	25	8
Orbital floor	9	3
Ala major	9	3
Lamina cribrosa (ethmoid)	8	3
Canalis opticus	5	2
Inferior orbital fissure	2	1

After passing through the orbital wall, the foreign body can enter various structures [137], such as the sinus frontalis, sinus maxillaris, sinus ethmoidalis, sinus sphenoidalis, nasal cavities, opposite orbit, pterygo-palatine fossa and finally, the most important, intracranial penetration can occur.

In our series, the frontal lobe was injured most frequently (41%), (including 37% abscesses, 44% contusions and 13% hematomas).

Yamaguchi *et al.* [153] as cited by Nakayama *et al.* [65] have stated that, in 63% of their cases of TIPI, frontal lobe injury occurred; a larger percentage than we found.

A description of an unusual cranio-orbital penetrating injury may be added; that is, a reverse penetration from inside the skull into the orbit, where a long metal rod entered the frontal lobe from the right fronto-temporal site to exit through the left orbit and upper eyelid [154].

PERFORATION THROUGH THE ORBITAL ROOF

As early as 1895, De Nobele [62] wrote that perforation through the orbital floor was very rare, while perforation through the orbital roof was common, especially at a location several millimeters in front of the foramen optimum. This happened for example in the case described by Anderson *et al.* [93]. Occasionally, the dura seems to be intact during surgical exploration in a case of radiological confirmed orbital roof perforation [155].

Greig [9] also suggested that the majority of traversing perforations occur through the roof of the eye socket. Miller *et al.* [108] reported that 71% of perforations enters through the orbital roof, 10% via the SOF and 5% through the lamina cribrosa. In our series, 50% of perforations entered through the orbital roof; thus, penetration frequently occurs in an upward direction.

Coqueret [20] had already described in 1905 the "mouvement de recul instinctif" (instinctive recoil). As a threatening object approaches the face, a defensive reflex causes the head to be thrown back [9], thus increasing the angle between the object and the orbital roof [47]. Thus, the object can no longer proceed to the back of the eye socket as easily, but will tend to perforate the orbital roof. The object's direction of approach is also significant; for example, in a fall trauma the head can be forced into retroflexion [2, 24, 150] and as a consequence, the direction of approach changes to upwards.

Fracture of the orbital roof or lamina cribrosa is, surgically speaking, a complicated comminutive impression fracture with bone fragments pushed inwards into the cerebrum [43]. Intracranial bone fragments are associated with an increased risk of infection [50] and should be removed. The immediate medial proximity of the nasal sinuses and the thin wall separating them (lamina papyracea) increases the risk of additional infection when this wall is damaged. Pathogens can also reach the injured brain tissue directly from the penetrating object itself, from the perforated skin or, later, by hematogenous infection.

From his study of traversing wounds of the orbit, Greig [9] concluded that there are important clinical consequences associated with either perforation of the orbital roof or through the SOF. According to him, the former traversing wounds initially appear to be trivial but later prove to be fatal. The frontal lobe can sustain an injury without initial symptoms if there is no rapid progressive expansive space-occupying lesion present, such as an increasing hematoma. Penetrations through the SOF, on the other hand, appear serious at the outset but recovery is possible, albeit with neurological defects.

Birch-Hirsfeld [110] argued against Greig's view: according to him, perforations through the SOF often prove to be fatal.

In this series, we found mortality to be twice as high (33%) for orbital roof injuries as for injuries through the SOF (15%). As expected, orbital roof penetration was frequently associated with frontal lobe damage (80% in this patient series) (Figure 26). Occasionally, direct injury of the internal capsule (6%) or the brainstem (4%) occurred, and even the sinus cavernosus could be injured, depending on the penetrating object's direction. Meningitis developed often (32%); temporary or chronic CSF leakage occurred in 14% of these cases.

A fracture of the back of the orbital roof and the upper rim of the canalis opticus could extend to the sphenoidal plane and the object could reach the hypothalamus and even the opposite lateral ventricle [156].

Diabetes insipidus appeared in 4.5%.

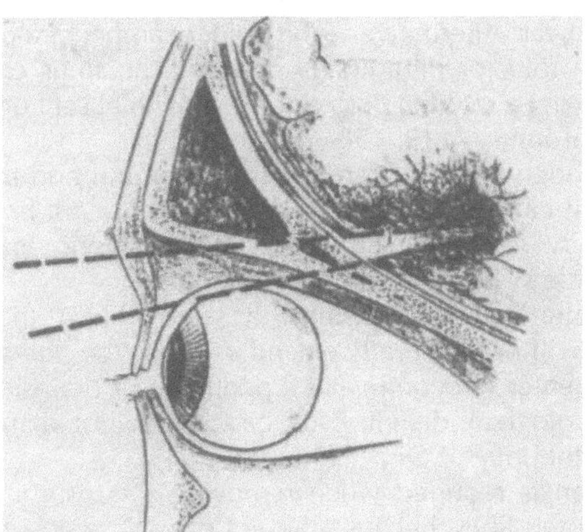

Figure 26 Structures damaged by a vertically directed transorbital stab

PENETRATION VIA THE SUPERIOR ORBITAL FISSURE (SOF)

In 1973, Merritt *et al.* [109] described a patient suffering from penetration through the SOF, according to him the fourth case presented in literature. However, this penetration path had already been published in 1834 by Scott [33 case 1] and in 1888 by Morrant Baker [7 case 2], and later by many others.

The SOF is an important point of entry into the intracranial space by orbit-penetrating objects [6]. In this patient series, penetration occurred via the SOF in 30%. Curiously enough, Duke-Elder [8, p. 443] does not even mention the possibility of intracranial penetration through the SOF but does accept penetration through the canalis opticus.

When the diameter of the penetrating object is somewhat larger than the opening of the SOF, a small, sometimes hard to find, fracture of the upper rim of the SOF (ala minor) may occur [7 case 2, 9]. A fracture of the ala major is possible given more thrust power and a penetrating object with a larger diameter [142].

Theoretically, the SOF can be reached most easily via the medial orbit as it is most accessible and open there for penetrating objects (Chapter 7).

In the current series, however, no clear distinction could be made: penetration through the medial part of the eye socket involved perforation through the SOF in 39% of cases and penetration through the lateral eye socket even more often, 48%. Penetration of the SOF through the lateral eye socket is thus certainly possible, probably due to the deflecting influence of the medial orbital wall [157] (Figure 27), or to sliding along the lateral wall.

An approximately horizontally entering agent, penetrating through the SOF, can reach the sinus cavernosus and the internal carotid artery medially or the temporal lobe laterally, depending on the direction and the force of the penetrating object. Alternatively, the object can penetrate deeply extradurally (in a dura fold) or intradurally between the sinus cavernosus and the temporal lobe deep into the posterior fossa, with absent or only minimal findings of clinical injury [139, 158–160].

Penetration through the SOF can remain extradural and the penetrating object, although it can be palpated [12, case 6] may not be found during exploratory surgery [72, 139, 158, 161]. With a more upward directed object, the ventricle system can be penetrated [62].

Given the anatomical relationships, it seems likely that penetration through the SOF will not generally extend as far as the contralateral hemisphere but could enter the contralateral peduncle or brainstem, producing homolateral neurological deficit. Nor can the hypothalamus be easily reached through the intact SOF.

Special attention is required when removing a transorbital penetrating twig stuck fast in the SOF, because the act of pulling it out may strip off the bark, leaving part of it *in situ* [19].

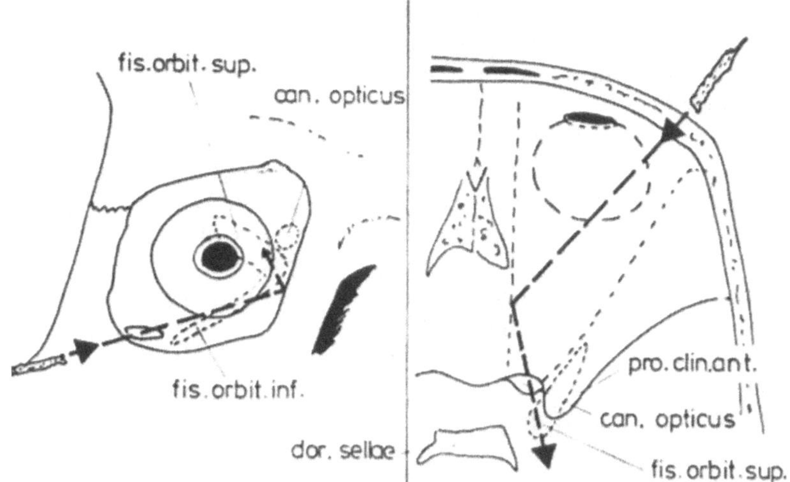

Figure 27 Foreign body deflected by the medial orbital wall, penetrating the SOF. Anatomical sketch of the orbit in frontal (left) and axial view demonstrating the pathomechanism of the injury

In this series, injuries were found at the following sites after penetration through the SOF:

Temporal lobe in 35%,
Brainstem in 34%,
Sinus cavernosus in 31%.

As expected, no frontal lobe injury was found. The brainstem can be easily reached via the basal cisterns following penetration through the SOF. The overall mortality associated with penetration through the SOF was 15%.

Sometimes an author claims that penetration occurred through the orbital roof, whereas the case history suggests penetration through the SOF [162], or the description mentions penetration through the CO while it clearly refers to penetration through the SOF [143].

PERFORATION THROUGH THE CANALIS OPTICUS (CO)

The CO represents a potential, but rarely seen, route of penetration. In 1998, 2 cases, caused by a chopstick, were published by Matsumoto *et al.* [23]. They found no previous reports in the English-language literature of this occurrence. However, in this series, 5 patients were described in the literature before 1998; only 2 suffered penetration via this route. Three of these 5 patients died; the 2 patients of Matsumoto *et al.* survived. A single report [142] referred to the CO as "the most common site of entry into the cranium" citing Duffy and Bandari [116], who wrote that "according to the literature" (unspecified), penetration often occurred through the CO. However, among Duffy's own patients, 5 of 6 cases of penetration involved the orbital roof.

The homolateral temporal lobe cannot be injured when the CO remains intact and unfractured. The latter is only 5 mm in diameter and has relatively strong walls. It is most accessible for midline directed objects, approaching from laterally below [140], in contrast to entry into the SOF. Penetration through the CO will irrevocably damage the optic nerve and, if continued across the midline, may seriously injure the hypothalamus [141 case 2] or enter the fossa interpeduncularis [77].

THE CONTRALATERAL INJURY

Penetrating objects with a general direction from lateral to medial can follow the strong lateral orbital wall, which forms an angle of 45° with the sagittal plane, and cause a contralateral injury, crossing the midline after perforating the laminae papyracea and cribrosa [1, 2]. Scarfo *et al.* [50], Unger and Umbach [59], McClure and Gardner [16 case 4], Gossman [163] and Morrant Baker [7 case 1] have described such cases.

Penetration through the medial canthus in an upwards and medially directed way can also perforate the ethmoid, cross the midline and cause a bilateral frontal lobe injury with intracerebral hematoma. The subsequent permanent complications can include a serious frontal syndrome due to a bifrontal lesion [78 case 1].

Crossing the midline can lead to injury to the hypothalamus, with severe associated symptoms like disturbances of consciousness, hyperthermia, diabetes insipidus, etc. A penetrating object crossing the midline via the ethmoid can also pass through the sinus sphenoidalis and through the clivus ending in the contralateral cerebello-pontine angle [74].

The foreign body does not always reach the contralateral side; sometimes its point is stuck in the sphenoid or clivus [105, 128, 164].

In this series, the midline was crossed in 39 patients (9%), 14 of whom died. Thirteen patients became comatose immediately, 4 of them temporarily. Five patients developed diabetes insipidus.

PERFORATION OF THE ORBITAL FLOOR

This does occur (in both directions), but rarely [7 case 12, 99, 165–170]. The sinus maxillaris can be reached through the orbital side of the orbital floor [7 case 12, 99, 165]. Through the back wall of the sinus maxillaris, the pterygo-palatine fossa can be reached, or the pharynx wall through the ethmoid, even as far as the anterior cervical spine without noticeable defects [167, 171]; the foreign object can even be palpable subcutaneously in the neck [168, 172]. This is thus an extracranial juxtabasal course. The naso-pharynx can be reached through the medial wall of the sinus maxillaris [94].

Perforation through the inferior orbital fissure [IOF] is rarely reported [144, 173]. According to De Nobele [68], both the IOF and the foramen rotundum are rarely injured by a penetrating agent as the convexity of the orbital floor just before the IOF and foramen rotundum prevents this. The pterygo-palatine fossa can be reached directly through the IOF [144]. Very rarely, perforation occurs through the sinus maxillaris, then subsequently through the orbital floor and roof, ending in the frontal lobe [50 case 2].

PERFORATION THROUGH THE ALA MAJOR

This is a rare injury, always involving a fracture. Although Duke-Elder [137] stated that, "The orbital walls may be fractured, *usually* (my italics) the frontal wing of the sphenoid", this is not so: fractures of the orbital roof occur far more frequently. The ala major bone is quite thick and considerable force is needed for perforation. An arrow shot from a compound bow would have sufficient force, as would a thrust with a garden cane [107].

The upper medial part of the ala major bone, bordering on the SOF, is somewhat thinner and thus easier to fracture and to perforate, leading to penetration into the temporal lobe [40, 107, 174].

Direct penetration through the lamina cribrosa or the ethmoid occurs with transnasal perforating injuries [64, 175, 176–180]; see also Chapter 17 of this volume.

A few cases have been described in the literature where the foreign body passed through one orbit and the ethmoid to reach the other orbit [20 case 48, 155 case 3, 181–183].

9

Clinical presentation and initial evaluation

The diagnosis of transorbital intracranial penetrating injury (TIPI) can be suggested by the presentation of a displaced eyeball, limitations in eye movement, protrusion of fat, blindness, etc. [8], which can be partially obscured by concurrent eyelid swelling, ecchymosis and chemosis.

Low-velocity orbital puncture wounds, however, often appear to be small innocent superficial puncture wounds, resulting from a simple injury, as attested by many authors [e.g. 1, 8, 14, 18, 78, 184] (Figure 28). Due to this apparent insignificance of the wound, the attending physician may be misled.

In this series, 14% did not have an injury to the eyelid; instead, perforation occurred through the conjunctiva. In 49%, only a small wound (<1 cm) was found; in 16% it was larger, while in 20% the size was not noted.

In addition, the eyeball is rarely injured. In this series, the eyeball remained intact in 74% and was damaged in 12% (in 14% not specified).

There may be no injury to the orbital structures [158] nor perforation wounds of the eyelids [97]. In these cases, the foreign body has taken a transorbital route through the fornix of the conjunctiva or via the canthus, between the eyelids [13, 97, 185].

The penetrating object may be absent, either because it was a fixed external object or because the victim, the bystanders or the aggressor has removed it. Under these circumstances it is uncertain how deep the injury is or what path it took; but a deep penetration must always be suspected.

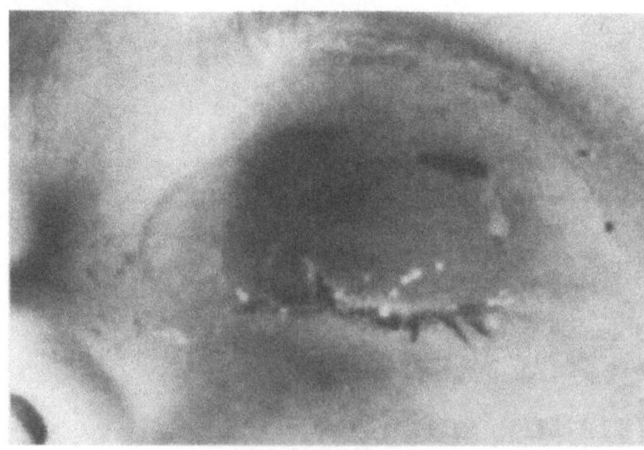

Figure 28 Child with a 1-cm laceration of the left upper eyelid

Multiple minor wounds in the face can distract attention away from a single dangerous deeply penetrating wound of the eyelid by suggesting that the "patient only fell on his face".

In this series, 25% of the patients presented for initial treatment with a penetrating object protruding from the eye socket. In 44%, the object was no longer present and had been totally removed, in 22% intraorbital and/or intracranial fragments remained, and, in 9%, no details were available.

The diagnosis of TIPI is often difficult to establish. Guthkelch [78] described 6 children with slight orbital wounds who later developed an intracranial infection. In only one child had intracranial penetration been suspected.

From the outset, an orbital wound must be considered a potentially serious deeply penetrating dangerous lesion, with parts broken off the penetrating object possibly still present along its course (orbital and/or intracranial). Such an injury must never be treated as an isolated lesion of the orbital content [10].

"All cases with penetrating wounds of the eyelids and orbit should be admitted to the hospital for observation" [8].

The absence of initial neurological findings does not preclude deep intracranial penetration [186]. It is important to carry out supplementary neuroradiological examination, such as conventional skull and orbit views, and CT and MR scans.

In practice, few orbital penetrating injuries extend intracranially, but the initial examination should assume that intracranial penetration has occurred until the opposite has been proven. Thus, the first examining physician must request supplementary radiological examinations, especially where children are involved.

Initially, there may be no cerebral symptoms [e.g. 114 case 1] present, particularly if penetration has occurred through the orbital roof with injury to the frontal lobe [e.g. 78 in 5 out of 6 cases] or through the SOF with injury to the temporal lobe; even the vision may be unaffected. In the frontal and temporal lobe, there may be a silent injury with a symptom-free interval, unless a large hematoma develops or extensive injury exists. This symptom-free interval is very misleading – analogous to the symptom-free interval with an epidural hematoma – and therefore dangerous for the patient. The doctor can easily feel that "everything has turned out all right".

In the current series, 33% of the patients had a symptom-free interval, usually lasting between 1 and 14 days (41%):

1–24 h:	16%
1–14 d:	41%
2–8 weeks:	21.6%
2–8 months:	10.3%
5–30 years:	11.1%

Penetration of the hypothalamus or brainstem immediately produces obvious and alarming symptoms. In this series, diabetes insipidus developed in 11 cases (temporary in 2) of whom 7 died.

Occasionally, temporary cerebral symptoms appear immediately after the injury, such as a short loss of consciousness, confusion or aphasia, signifying intracranial extension of the transorbital injury [10, 187].

In this series, 34% of the patients showed immediate symptoms. (In one third of the total group, it was unclear when the symptoms began.) These acute symptoms included a temporary loss of consciousness, semicoma and coma in 39%; vomiting and some clouding of consciousness as drowsiness, sopor, disorientation, delirium, or agitation in 34%; hemiplegia in 18%; and seizures in 3%.

Other symptoms were neck-stiffness, ocular nerve injury, gaze palsy, hypo-dysesthesies, cerebellar symptoms, etc.

On the other hand, a small wooden foreign body lodged in the SOF may produce only a low-grade fever [157].

A TIPI may heal without producing clinical symptoms. In some publications, the author does not always consider the possibility of an asymptomatic TIPI. From the length of the removed object, however, it is certain that penetration did occur. Unfortunately, intracranial penetration is often only eventually diagnosed when serious neurological symptoms appear. Early diagnosis could have prevented these complications. A slight 'conjunctiva wound' can result in death 3 weeks later due to the development of a brain abscess [188]. Miller *et al.* [108] found, in their series, that one third of the patients evidenced immediate symptoms, one third developed problems within 1 week, while the remainder remained asymptomatic for 2 weeks to 13 years.

10
Physical examination

The first step, of course, is a general physical examination to establish whether the patient is in a life-threatening condition. If so, measures to alleviate this situation have the highest priority, such as airway check, hypoxia prevention, ensuring hemodynamic stability, preventing shock, looking for other serious injuries, etc. These important matters will not be discussed here.

HISTORY

The examination begins with taking an adequate history and/or hetero-anamnesis [60, 150] while keeping in mind the primary golden rule: exercise a high degree of suspicion. Wounds of the orbit should always suggest the possibility of a deep intracranial penetration. If suspected, immediate hospital admission is recommended for further investigation and observation [185].

Reconstruction of the accident should be attempted in order to determine:

1. What is the nature of the penetrating object? How long was it? Was the object made of wood and, if so, was the wood dry or green? (In Chapter 11 on Neuroimaging, the significance of this question for CT and MR diagnostics is discussed.)
2. How deep was the penetration; estimate the direction of penetration [24]. Assume that the perforation probably went deeper than the witnesses of the accident report [11].
3. Is there any remaining piece or even multiple fragments of the penetrating object still in the wound? Even if the object has already been removed from the orbit, it should be assumed that pieces have remained *in situ* [43], especially if the object has broken off [184]. Try to get hold of the object and examine it carefully [24, 150] to see whether it is complete or not.

History taking is often unreliable or impossible, especially with children. Occasionally, children keep silent about the accident because they are afraid of punishment [155 case 1, 189 cases 1 and 2]. Always suspect that there might be a non-accidental cause of the trauma: (attempted) suicide or aggression with possibly fatal consequences could be involved [190].

Alcohol or drug intoxication hampers history taking and further examination. There is the danger that alterations of consciousness are ascribed to intoxication, thus missing the signs and symptoms of an intracranial complication.

Sometimes the history is unreliable because the injury happened so quickly that the victim does not fully grasp what occurred [49]. It is also possible that symptoms appear so late after the injury that the patient has forgotten about the injury in the meantime or does not mention it because he does not see the connection between the present symptoms and the preceding injury. However, at operation or at autopsy, the true nature of the symptoms may be established [175, 78 case 5, 191]. A CSF fistula or recurrent meningitis lasting for years may finally lead to the true diagnosis [192].

If the penetrating object (pencil, branch, rod, knife) is still in the orbit when the patient is admitted to the ED, the prevailing urge is to pull it out; indeed, this has often already been done by the victim him- or herself or bystanders. Although, admittedly, this may have no repercussions, it is better not to remove the object because severe complications might occur [55]. Simply pulling out a transorbital intracranially penetrating foreign body can be very risky [193]. As early as 1818 Demours[1] described removal of a foreign body in a 10-year-old child leading to fatal hemorrhage [19]. In 1872, La Force reported a case of a 10-year-old boy who died immediately after pulling a 10-cm-long piece of wood out of his eye socket [38].

In this series, the mortality of patients presenting after the foreign body had already been removed was twice that of patients presenting with the foreign body still *in situ*. The point of the penetrating object can act as a sort of 'tampon', its removal thus leading to fatal bleeding [194]. Reactive removal of a knife penetrating deeply in the eye socket can lead to a worse prognosis [53, 194], as the knife – often being stuck – must be turned and jiggled to pry it loose when it is jammed, thus producing more injury. However, a shallow penetration probably results in less injury even if the blade moves during removal.

The object should be removed via the orbit only after a detailed radiological investigation has shown whether craniotomy with intracranial supervising of important nearby structures (e.g. blood vessels) is necessary. Immediate removal has another disadvantage as it is more difficult to ascertain the direction of the path of the penetrating object [155] although modern neuroimaging may be able to shed light on this.

OPHTHALMOLOGIC EXAMINATION

Even for an apparently trivial orbital wound, an exhaustive ophthalmologic examination is the next step required, keeping in mind that "intracranial

[1] Maladies des yeux, 1818, in Graefe–Saemisch Bd 6, p. 638; 268

extension is often not suspected when an orbital wound is examined" [71]. A slight eyelid wound can be difficult to spot if there is concurrent eyelid swelling, hematoma or edema, subconjunctival bleeding, chemosis, ecchymosis, proptosis, etc. masking the site of entry [71]. In addition, folds in the eyelid skin can hide a small puncture wound. Occasionally, no injury can be found [9]. Transconjunctival entry of a foreign body may be obscured by chemosis [60], but can also be invisible in and by itself [71]. A small eyelid wound or conjunctiva injury heals within a week, leaving a barely visible scar. However, foreign particles still present deep inside may remain unnoticed [175] for a long time due to lack of clinical signs [136]. Much later, a fistula may arise or deeply situated (anaerobic) bacteria may produce symptoms [10].

By simply everting the eyelid, a defect in the conjunctiva may be revealed, which will require further investigation [90]. If orbital fat is evident in the wound, then the orbital septum has been penetrated and there is a serious risk of deep penetration with pieces of the object left behind [60].

Occasionally, a short-lived mild leakage of CSF through the puncture opening is the only indication of TIPI [16 case 1, 24 case 2, 78 case 6]. The loss of CSF through an orbital injury, however, can also be persistent [195]. The nature of the fluid can be established by measuring the glucose content, as CSF contains at least 30 mg/ml glucose. Glucose oxidative paper tests are too inaccurate for this purpose [71]. Concurrent hemorrhaging or a severe eye injury can mask CSF loss but should not be missed.

Children with apparently minor orbital injury, in particular, must be examined closely for evidence of deep penetration as their orbital roof is very thin and easily perforated.

Severe eye socket symptoms, such as swelling, ecchymosis, hematoma and proptosis, can obfuscate an intracranial penetration and mild CSF loss.

Due to the neurological implications and failure to appreciate an afferent pupil defect, no pupil-dilating agents should be employed during ophthalmologic examination.

Immediate and complete loss of vision generally indicates irrecoverable damage to n2, but sometimes vision can be restored [196]. Fundus examination will reveal whether the optical nerve is damaged posteriorly (normal fundus) or anteriorly (anemic fundus) from the point of entry of the ophthalmic artery.

The eyeball often remains intact (74% of our series) if the object is thin. The firm sclera resists a certain amount of force and the eyeball can be easily pushed aside in the orbital fat, opening up a route to the posterior orbit. The seriousness of a (low-velocity) injury depends on the size, direction, nature and force of the penetrating object, the angle of penetration, the site of entry, the depth of the wound and the orbit's architecture. The ED physician and the ophthalmologist are of prime importance when the patient is admitted, but the ultimate care of a transorbital injury will be supplied by a team consisting of an ophthalmologist, a neurosurgeon, a neuroradiologist, and possibly an ENT specialist and a plastic surgeon. The ophthalmologist should remain involved in the care in order to supervise the orbital side of the injury, preventing unnecessary loss of eye function [5].

NEUROLOGICAL EXAMINATION

A detailed and repeatedly conducted neurological examination, including the Glasgow Coma Scale (GCS), is essential when intracranial injury is suspected. The site and extent of the intracranial and possible vascular injury determine the onset of acute neurological symptoms.

In a number of cases, hemiplegia appears immediately, due to injury to the internal capsule or peduncle (18%). A homolateral hemiplegia suggests midline crossing with contralateral injury of the internal capsule or peduncle [197]. However, normal neurological parameters do not rule out a transorbital brain lesion: a frontal or temporal lobe injury can initially be asymptomatic, and an object can penetrate through the SOF as far as the posterior cranial fossa without producing symptoms (Figure 29).

An initial carefully conducted neurological examination may reveal a subtle symptom, such as a horizontal gaze paresis in the undamaged eye [185] or slight cerebellar coordination disturbances [75], clearly identifying a deep unsuspected penetration.

Loss of nerve control of the eye muscles (n3, n4, n6) arising 1 week after the injury may indicate the development of a traumatic aneurysm of the carotid artery in the sinus cavernosus [198]. Loss of n6 function, appearing 3 months after injury, can suggest a carotid–cavernosus fistula [199: 'symptôme précoce', precocious symptom]. Bizarre brainstem symptoms should not be ascribed to a subarachnoid hemorrhage as they may result from a deep penetration [56].

When the patient shows meningeal irritation, lumbar puncture – only performed after a space-occupying lesion has been ruled out – can establish the presence of blood and/or infection. Finding blood in the CSF is proof of intracranial penetration [187]. Previously, air insufflation was used during lumbar puncture, but this can lead to a fatal hemorrhage when a thrombus in the perforated wall of the sinus cavernosus is dislodged [76, 200].

Neurological supervision should not be limited to one initial examination. Continuous careful monitoring is necessary as a drop in the GCS, and confusion, irritability, nuchal rigidity, CSF leakage, etc. are all important signs of intracranial penetration. An extensive neuroradiological examination is essential, especially if the history is fragmentary. In Chapter 11, on Neuroimaging, this is discussed in detail.

Wound cultures will give an indication of the bacterial flora already present in the wound. Tetanus antitoxin and antibiotics (Chapter 13) should

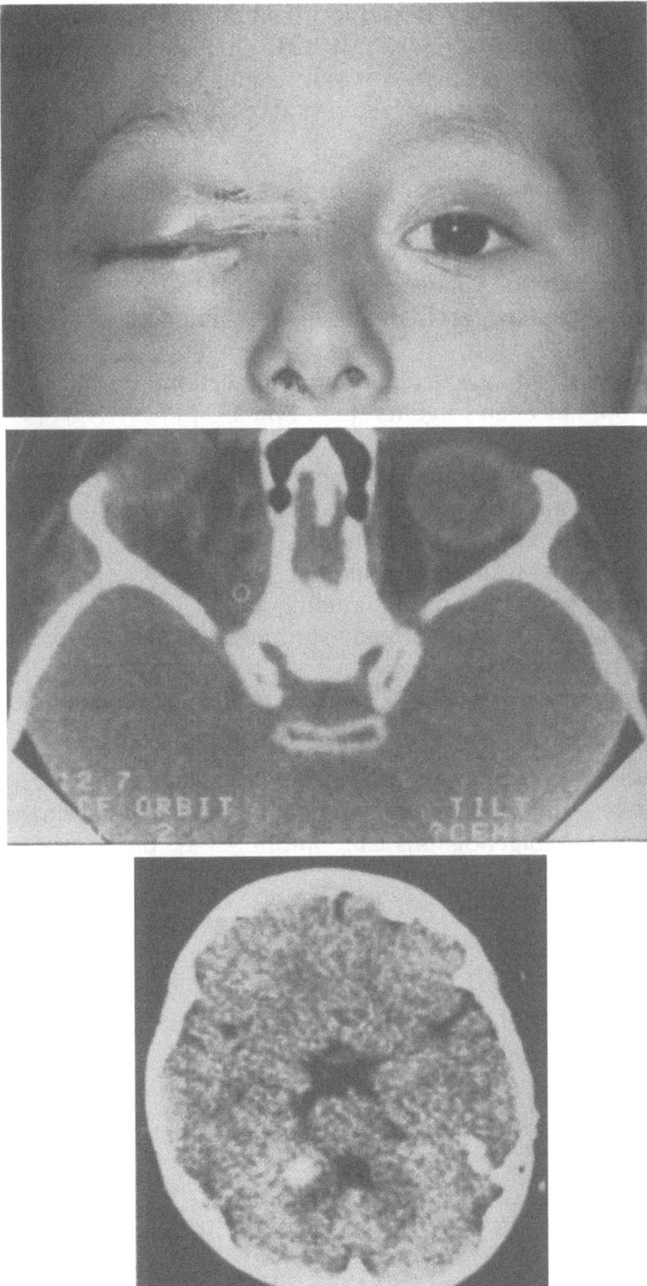

Figure 29 Young girl with TIPI, struck with an arrow through the right upper lid. Complete ophthalmoplegia and loss of visual acuity. Orbital emphysema and soft-tissue mass in the posterior orbit. Hematoma in the posterior fossa adjacent to the fourth ventricle. Apart from mildly reduced muscular tone, no other neurologic abnormalities

be given to the patient. In the earlier literature, tetanus was described in association with this injury [10, 110, 201] but is rarely seen nowadays because of widespread prophylaxis with tetanus toxoid.

Let us summarize a number of factors that could obstruct early recognition of TIPI:

1. Deep penetration may not be suspected and the injury treated as a minor one.
2. Only a slight or no eyelid wound (fornix perforation) from which the penetrating object has already been removed.
3. A heavily swollen, ecchymotic eyelid hiding a small penetrating wound.
4. The history is incomplete (children, intoxication).
5. The trauma has been forgotten [e.g. 78 case 5].
6. No initial neurological symptoms (symptom-free interval).
7. Routine radiographs of the skull and orbits show no abnormalities.
8. A concurrent alcohol or drug intoxication obstructing not only history-taking but also further examination.
9. A large obvious wound elsewhere.
10. Absence of eyeball or/and optic nerve injury.
11. Blood in the CSF being incorrectly attributed to SAH due to an aneurysm or a 'traumatic tap'.
12. Signs of infection in the CSF leading to the incomplete diagnosis of meningitis [23].

To conclude this chapter, we quote from Bursick and Selker [202]: "The combination of a minor-appearing wound, unremarkable physical examination and normal roentgenograms can, unfortunately, prove fatal."

11 Neuroimaging

INDICATIONS

The radiological examination is a crucial element involved in the diagnosis and treatment of a transorbital injury because, in a large percentage of cases, the patient presents with a minor external injury (63%) and no initial cerebral symptoms. There is often a symptom-free interval before complications appear (33%), giving the illusion of no injury to the brain. Careful and repeated neurological examination sometimes shows early signs of a deep penetrating injury, but it should – at the slightest suspicion – always be combined with a thorough radiological examination. Even apparently innocent wounds of the eye socket must be considered for extensive radiological examination. This examination can diagnose and localize injury to the eyeball, the soft parts of the orbit, and/or the intracranial contents and ascertain the presence of fractures of the walls between the orbit and the neighboring structures. Remaining parts of the foreign body and any punched-in bone fragments can be found. Very important is the opportunity that modern neuroimaging provides for intracranial pathology analysis. Before considering surgical therapy, thorough detailed neuroimaging should be carried out, including angiography if indicated.

AVAILABLE METHODS

Orbital ultrasonography

Orbital ultrasonography is felt by most authors to have limited value [203, 204]. If available, the less-expensive standardized echography (combined use of standardized A scan and B scan) can be considered as a first-line investigation, requiring, however, specific expertise and technology not available in many hospitals [204]. The method cannot evaluate the entire orbit, especially not the apex. It is a time-consuming examination and the results depend on the examiner's experience. A negative result is inconclusive. It does not reveal intraorbitally situated wood surrounded by air [166] or foreign bodies smaller than 2 mm [203, 206]. Wooden foreign bodies as small as 2.5 mm in length can be effectively located by US [207] although it is difficult to perform if the patient is uncooperative. For the neurosurgeon, this examination does not yield information regarding intracranial complications. High-resolution ultrasound examination may give better results.

Conventional orbit and skull radiographs (anteroposterior, lateral, Caldwell, Waters, Rhese, submento–vertex views)

It is difficult to obtain a good image of the orbital walls, especially of the thin orbital roof, where intracranial penetration often occurs. Fractures are thus commonly missed, as attested in many case histories in the literature.

The study by Bard and Jarrett [12] concerning the initial standard radiograph is illuminating in this respect. Among 44 cases of transorbital penetration in the literature, 34 of whom underwent an initial radiological examination, he found "some evidence of penetration beyond the orbit" in 19 cases (56%). In 15 patients, the result was negative, while, in 10 patients, abnormalities were seen only on subsequent examination. In his own series of 9 cases, 8 underwent an initial radiological examination and in only one case was an injury of the orbital wall identified. In 30% of cases, no standard radiographic evidence of intracranial injury was present [178].

In this series, an initial (or somewhat delayed) radiological examination was performed in 52%. Of these, 41% showed no evidence of a fracture.

A 'normal' radiograph, therefore, cannot rule out the possibility of an orbital fracture and further examination is still indicated. Special methods, such as tomography and tangential views, may improve visualization [156], but are difficult to perform with confused and restless patients; in addition, radiation exposure is high.

In children, the orbital roof is particularly thin, and therefore it is easy to miss a perforation.

Small bone pieces from the orbital roof can be punched inward and are difficult to see on standard radiographs [13].

Perforation through the SOF or CO can occur without fracture. Occasionally, thin-section tomography will reveal only a widening of the SOF, which may indicate the presence of a (wooden) foreign body here [208]. It is important to note that under normal circumstances the left and right SOF are not exactly identical and can differ in width. Evidence of a fracture is often associated with more serious findings during surgery.

Radio-opaque foreign bodies, such as metal objects, are obviously easy to find, and their depth and intracranial localization can be estimated. However, it is important to consider that the object may have penetrated more deeply than apparent on the image. When retracting the head after a fall on a fixed and broken-off object (e.g. a car antenna) or when removing a ballpoint pen whose tip remains *in situ* [209], the foreign body may be retracted some distance, thus ending now more superficially. The real initial penetration was actually deeper.

These guidelines also apply to CT and MR examination, although the originally deeper penetration track is more likely to be shown.

This phenomenon may explain why a thrombosis of the carotid artery (probably due to an intima tear) is occasionally seen where surgical exploration did not reveal an external injury of the artery or even any direct contact between the penetrating object and the carotid artery [159, 193].

Low-density foreign bodies, such as plastic, glass and especially wood, may be missed. A pencil can be visualized due to its central graphite core and possibly a metal-based coating [114]. Lead-containing paint on a wooden foreign body can make it visible [210].

Injuries to the intraorbital or intracranial soft parts are beyond detection by conventional radiology.

Pneumocephalus, produced by a fracture in the walls of the paraorbital sinuses, is usually quickly noticed (more easily than the orbital fracture itself) and may be the only indication of a TIPI [106, 211]. Pneumocephalus may develop late and only become evident on repeated images during follow-up (2 weeks to 2 months, [106]).

Conventional radiological studies are thus nothing more than a superficial and maybe superfluous screening, leading only to avoidable and unwanted radiation exposure [212]. However, they rule out the presence of a metal foreign body, thus permitting MRI to be carried out.

Although there is frequently no obvious radiological abnormality (41%), of course it may be *clinically* evident that intracranial penetration has occurred.

CT IMAGING

The image in CT is built up from variations in tissue density and the density gradient between the foreign body and the tissue. CT has contributed significantly to the recognition and treatment of the frequently clinically obscure TIPI. It has become irreplaceable, as it reveals even totally unsuspected intracranial injury [213]. In addition, the orbital contents and their pathology, bone fractures and the presence of a foreign body are made evident.

With bone window views, CT is an ideal method to find fractures; even small fractures can be traced (Figure 30). Scans in the coronary plane show the orbital walls and the neighboring sinuses quite clearly. It is important to determine whether neighboring sinuses are perforated, thus carrying a higher risk of infection.

However, as mentioned, the absence of a fracture does not exclude an intracranially penetrating injury, as both the SOF and, more rarely, the CO can provide easy access to the intracranial space.

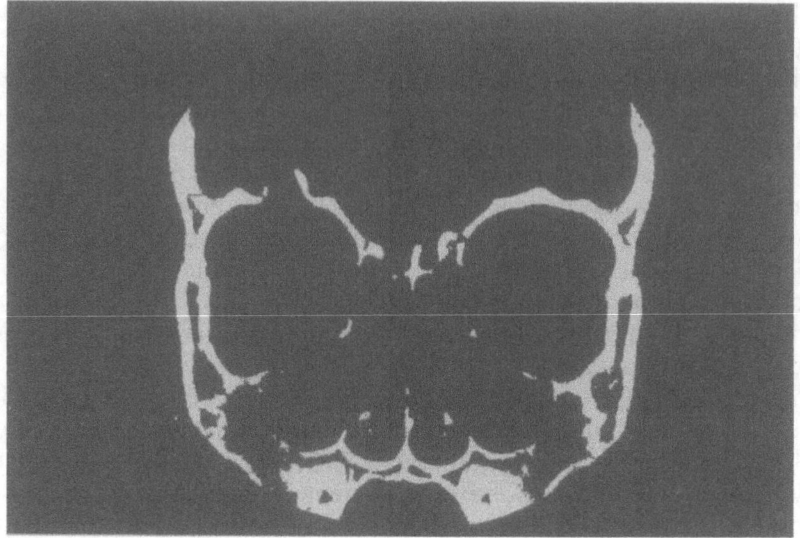

Figure 30 CT bone windows clearly show a displaced fracture of the orbital roof

Bone splinters and broken-off pieces of the foreign body can also be revealed, if necessary, by preparing thin slices (1.5–3 mm) in the axial and coronary planes.

The orientation of the foreign body to the beam direction is very significant. If its long axis is parallel to the CT scanner rays, the foreign body may not show up due to averaging.

Preparing three-dimensional reconstructions may give additional information [52]. The presence of air intracranially is immediately evident; even 0.5 ml is visible [214] and this is proof of intracranial penetration. If intracerebral gas is present, the presence of gas-forming bacteria must also be considered [215]. Subarachnoid hemorrhage is made visible, calling for angiography.

A large metal object situated intracranially (e.g. a knife) can hinder the interpretation of the scans due to the production of an artifact [194].

The path of the penetrating object – often seen as a low-density track in the brain [216] with small hemorrhages – can give an estimate of the extent of tissue damage and the potential neurological pathology. Punched-in bone fragments, hemorrhaging and abscesses can be revealed, along with the foreign object or any remaining pieces of it. The condition of the ventricle system can be evaluated. The presence of a small area of high density in the traumatized region could be a foreign body rather than a calcium deposit [217].

One great advantage of CT is its swiftness, preventing motion artifacts like eye movements.

Its disadvantages include:

1. Vascular injury cannot be demonstrated directly [218], but contrast enhancement can show a carotid–cavernosus fistula (CCF) or a traumatic aneurysm.
2. CT poorly portrays small foreign bodies with a density more or less similar to that of the surrounding tissue. In particular, wooden objects are notorious in this respect. Wood splinters easily and recognizing multiple small pieces of wood is difficult with CT. Neuroimaging of wooden foreign objects will be treated separately in detail below.

However, CT is cost-effective and utilizes a smaller radiation dose than orbital tomography.

The sensitivity of CT can be increased by [128, 219]:

1. Using multiple window settings, i.e. soft-tissue as well as bone window settings are helpful in distinguishing structures of similar density, such as low-density foreign bodies.
2. Preparing thin scans (1–1.5–3 mm) in the axial, coronary and possibly tangential planes [220].
3. Image reversal sometimes enhances fracture details [219].
4. Three-dimensional reconstructions.
5. Using contrast to enhance reactive tissue surrounding the foreign body.

In the initial phase of every orbital penetrating injury, a CT scan should be performed to determine the condition of the orbit and to exclude or uncover any intracranial penetration. It is reasonable to repeat the CT study after 1–2 weeks to reveal any intracerebral abscess formation [194]. If the score on the Glasgow Coma Scale drops, a repeat scan becomes a matter of urgency [98].

CT AND WOODEN FOREIGN BODIES

The transorbital penetrating wooden object presents a special problem. In 1993, Ginsberg *et al.* [221] called CT analysis of this sort of injury a 'pitfall'. Recent review articles regarding the radiological assessment of trauma and foreign bodies of the eye and orbit (1996 [222]) or the current use of orbital CT in the MR era (1998 [28]) barely mention the problems associated with the neuroimaging of intraorbital and/or intracranial wooden foreign bodies.

The CT image is affected by the dimensions and the physical density (g/cm^3) of the wood, which in turn depends on its water content (green or dry wood) and the type (hard or softwood) [56]. The density of wood is a multifactoral phenomenon [223].

In addition, coatings or infection and the presence of reactive tissue can influence the CT image. The density of wood varies widely and can overlap

Table 3 Density values of wood

Minimum (hu)	Maximum (hu)	Year	Reference	Notes
−552	+54	1977	[225]	Wet wood
−350	−150	1980	[180]	
−310		1984	[226]	
−618	+23	1987	[227]	
−405	−126	1988	[228]	Literature: −600 to +27
−461	−88	1988	[146]	
−999	−67	1990	[229]	
−461	+68	1992	[178]	
−610	+23	1995	[203]	
−550	+289	1995	[223]	
−600	+130	1997	[212]	

with that of the surrounding orbital or intracranial tissue and even bone, making identification difficult [224]. Various authors have given density values derived from (*in-vitro*) investigations (Table 3). For example, a chopstick can have a density of −108 hu [79]. In a transorbital injury, the wooden foreign object is often dry, with a low density (e.g. −496 hu) as a result of trapped air and its cellulose composition [221]. Thus, using standard soft-tissue CT levels and window settings, the wood will be perceived as 'air', especially if fractures are involved [224]. Many such cases are described in the literature [e.g. 213]. This can lead to wood being missed [11, 152, 230, 231].

If soft-tissue window settings only are used, dry wood will appear as 'air' [77, 213, 220, 221, 223, 226–228, 232, 233].

In 1990, Glatt *et al.* [229] reported a review of CT studies of nine patients injured by wooden foreign bodies. In three cases, the object was not found. Nevertheless, he feels that we can be too pessimistic concerning CT's ability to detect wood. More modern equipment can achieve this if appropriate window settings are used.

A number of factors facilitate identification of dry wood:

1. The contours and geometric form of a wooden foreign body are generally elongated and sharply outlined [114, 167, 220, 224]. It appears as a low-density structure with sharp borders [234].
2. The size does not change at follow-up.
3. The density can increase due to water absorption [223].
4. Gradually, surrounding granulation tissue will appear as a reaction, increasing density.
5. Density values of −600 hu strongly suggest wood [228], although small wood fragments can be missed [204] or, due to the partial volume effect, cannot be distinguished from air [228, 229].

6. Variable window width settings should be used [166, 220], i.e. not just soft-tissue settings but also wide bone settings [126, 220, 229, 233]; using standard settings alone, wood can be missed.
7. Wide bone settings may reveal the reticulate matrix of wood [221, 233].

The density of dry wood can change from low to high values (e.g. from −599 hu to +68 hu [228]) over a number of weeks (occasionally after 8 days [81]) due to water absorption – which varies according to wood type [221] – and to a foreign body reaction around the wood or possibly through calcium precipitation in the wood [234]. Water immersion can alter the image even within 48 h by increasing the density [235], making identification in the orbit or intracranially even more difficult as the values approach those of the surrounding tissue [178, 233]. Thus, wood becomes more difficult to identify over time. Before complete saturation is accomplished, water uptake, from outside the piece of wood to inside, may cause an identifiable image of inhomogenity [212].

Drying out of the wood *in-vitro* leads to a reduced density [228]. Density analysis can help distinguish between dry wood and air. Air has a value of −1022 hu, while dry wood, e.g. from a pencil, can measure −539 hu [144, 229]. With a wide window of 1000 hu and a level of −500 hu, wood can be shown to have a somewhat higher density than air [166]. Surrounding infection or granuloma [236] and coatings of metal-based paint can suggest the presence of a wooden foreign body [151]. The location of wood along surfaces with varying radiodensities, such as the orbital floor or a soft-tissue/air interface [232], can hinder its discovery [203, 237].

After removal of a wooden foreign body, the tissue shows the usual postoperative changes, making it difficult to discover any remaining pieces of wood *in situ* [178, 218], leading to possible reinfection [238, 239]. In practice, the radiologist is faced with the difficult question of whether wooden fragments are still present after operation [239].

A pencil has various densities as it consists of a wooden shell around a graphite core; in principle, this is a soft-tissue mass surrounding a dense core [160], which can measure +235 hu [144]. The density of a pencil's wood ranges from −175 [180] to −440/−500 hu [238] or even −539 hu [144]. The graphite core appears as a dense linear fragment, sometimes bordered by signs of chronic osteomyelitis or benign reactive osteitis [240]. T1 MR imaging of a pencil can produce a signal artifact, causing the object to appear larger than its actual size. This is called the 'blooming' artifact and is caused by the presence of both iron and magnesium in the object, inducing a local magnetic field around it and thereby increasing the apparent size of the pencil lead [241].

Therefore, if CT imaging shows 'air' after an orbital injury or TIPI, we must suspect that this 'air' shadow, especially if it is linear, could be a wooden foreign object [212, 228, 232] and its density must be measured [228].

If necessary, additional CT examination (contrast media, dynamic or delayed contrast-enhanced scans, thin section CT, coronal, tangential and sagittal cuts, angling of axial cuts, reconstruction etc.) can be performed [146, 178].

CT can also miss a foreign body made of plastic [97].

FURTHER RESEARCH INTO DETECTION OF WOODEN FOREIGN BODIES BY CT AND MRI

As the identification of wood presents difficulties in CT and MRI, much research has concentrated on (partly *in-vitro*) studies with both methods.

We summarize the principal results:

Healy, 1980 [180]: CT can distinguish wood in the brain from the surrounding tissue, but the wooden foreign body looks like air. Wood, surrounded by bone, can be identified using narrow window settings because of its low density.

Tate and Cupples, 1981 [204]: small wood fragments are not detected with CT.

Kaiser *et al.*, 1983 [238]: by using very narrow window settings, a wooden foreign body (pencil) can be made visible with clarity.

Jooma *et al.*, 1984 [226]: the first reported CT demonstration of intracranial penetration by wood, misinterpreted as air, was probably made by Lunsford *et al.*, 1977 [213].

Myllylä *et al.*, 1987 [227]: CT differentiation between wood and gas is problematical. Small wood fragments have proved undetectable. The density of wood varies from −618 to +23 hu.

Gückel, 1988 [228]: green wood has a higher density than dry wood and hardwood likewise a higher density than softwood. The ringed structure of wood can lead to a higher density value in the core, according to the type of wood and the degree of hydration. If a wooden foreign body is not recognized and thus remains *in situ*, the original difference in density between the wood and the surrounding reactive tissue will lessen with time as the wood absorbs water. Directly after the penetrating injury, CT can differentiate wood from air by density measurements.

Hansen *et al.*, 1988 [146]: dry wood can, depending on the type, have an average density of −461 to −88 hu. After soaking, all types of wood showed a higher density. Six types of wood, dry and wet, varied greatly in density, similar to the orbital, periorbital and intracranial tissues. Accurate foreign body content identification is not always possible.

Glatt *et al.*, 1990 [229]: carried out *in-vitro* investigations of wood with CT and MRI. Earlier authors reported absorption coefficients of −700 to +54 hu. Glatt *et al.* showed that larger pieces of dry wood had values between −984 and −356 hu and were thus hypodense to fat. The CT absorption coefficient of different types of wood varied from −999 to −67 hu, according to type, size and water content of the wood; most types of wood are hypodense to fat. Orbital fat has an absorption coefficient of approximately −100 hu. After 3 days of immersion in water, the density of plywood increased the most. Green wood had a density of −274 to −70 hu, with a window width of 1000 hu; it could be easily distinguished from a fat background. Types of wood such as pine and walnut appear as a hypodense core surrounded by denser rings.

The CT image of a pencil (a very dense inner core surrounded by a hypodense cortex) does not change after removal of the paint coating [151]. In this study, a wide window (up to 1000 hu) was optimal for detecting all but the smallest pieces of wood by distinguishing it from fat.

In clinical practice, however, it is better to work with multiple window settings because there are always complications hindering the evaluation, e.g. movement artifacts, hemorrhage, reactive tissue around the foreign body and possibly air.

Small pieces of wood have higher CT absorption coefficients and cannot be distinguished from small air bubbles with CT (partial volume averaging effect) nor with MRI. MRI was better at finding small pieces of wood in a vegetable fat background (chosen to simulate orbital fat).

Fallon *et al.*, 1992 [178]: wood has a density of −461 to +68 hu.

Phytinen *et al.*, 1995 [223]: the accuracy of CT depends on the density gradient between the foreign body and the surrounding tissue. A wooden foreign body can appear to have the same density as gas (pine −550 hu) or bone (ebony +289 hu). Wood clearly has a wide range of hu values and misinterpretation as gas still occurs.

Dalley, 1995 [233]: green wood, having a higher density than dry wood due to its greater water content, is more difficult to distinguish from the orbital and intracranial soft tissues by either CT or MRI [239]. Wide bone window settings usually reveal the striate internal architecture of wood, i.e. its reticulate matrix, distinguishing it from gas. However, if the wood has a density approaching that of fat, identification can be difficult.

MRI can be tried, as it is superior to CT in the detection of dry wood [77, 229, 232, 233]. However, both CT and MRI can miss green wood or rehydrated wood.

CT soft-tissue window settings (e.g. 350 hu width and 40 hu level), which reveal an 'air shadow' must not be used alone but bone window settings must also be used, e.g. 4000 hu width and 400 hu level; here the 'gas density' appears to be partly solid with a striate matrix, characteristic of dry wood. The wide bone settings (reconstructed twice, using a bone algorithm) serve to optimize edge definition and to distinguish air from wood or fat.

Ho *et al.*, 1996 [166]: wood can be distinguished from air by density analysis. Using a wide window of 1000 hu and level of −500 hu, it can be seen that wood has a somewhat higher density than air. The geometric contour of the wooden fragment(s) may allow them to be inferred.

McGuckin *et al.*, 1996 [224]: *in-vitro* experiments show that, for CT images, variations in window width and level are very important to differentiate wood from gas, fat and extracellular fluid. *In vitro,* MRI cannot differentiate dry wood or the bark of green wood from air or bone fragments. Fresh pine is slightly better seen on MR than CT. CT with optimal image contrast (using the proper window settings) can distinguish dry and green wood from air and bone and is thus the method of first choice. CT is also unaffected by metal and is cheaper, easier and faster than MRI.

MAGNETIC RESONANCE IMAGING

MR T1- and T2-weighted images cohere with the variations in the density of protons in the tissues and their relaxation times [232] and thus vary with the type of wood and its water content [233]. The method reproduces differences in signal intensity due to variations in the proton content of wood and surrounding tissue, thus producing an image of a wooden foreign body in the orbit and/or intracranially [239]. Dry wood has lower signal intensity than fat on T1-weighted images [233].

MRI has certain disadvantages:

1. Bone images are not optimal;
2. It cannot be used when a metallic foreign body is *in situ*;
3. More cooperation is required of the patient;
4. Scanning times are longer; thus, more movement artifacts may occur.

A selection of authors who have studied the problem of finding a wooden foreign body using MRI, is cited:

Wilson *et al.*, 1988 [242] found that dry wood (pine) could be identified by both CT and MRI, but CT revealed the shape of the foreign body better and characterized its composition. Their MR scanner, however, had technical limitations, such as a weak magnet and a large slice thickness. Dry wood produced a lower signal and a hypointense image compared with fat on T1-weighted MR images, which are better than T2-weighted images; both detection and localization were more difficult with T2-weighted images, probably because of the loss of signal intensity in the orbital fat.

Gückel, 1988 [228] felt that MRI, due to improved resolution, can show wood surrounded by granulation tissue because of the ringed aspect with a high-intensity core (the marrow) and a high-intensity bark. In this manner, both T1- and T2-weighted images can distinguish between granulomatous changes and gas accumulation, while CT could not reveal any hypodense structure at this stage. This varies, however, due to the extent of hydration and type of wood. MRI is therefore indicated for older injuries because it can sometimes reveal the ringed aspect of wood in spite of a granulomatous tissue reaction.

Green *et al.*, 1990 [232]: MRI can demonstrate wood situated intraorbitally. Initially, a wooden object in this location appears as air on CT scans, whereas T1-weighted images show the wooden foreign body as a well-delineated low-intensity lesion, suggestive of a foreign body. The presence of air does make interpretation difficult however.

Glatt *et al.*, 1990 [229] ascertained that, on MRI, all types of wood, even green wood, are hypointense to fat, making detection possible.

MRI studies of wood in a vegetable fat background (chosen to simulate orbital fat) showed that small pieces of wood produced hypointense images surrounded by an artifact with hyperintense spots, the so-called truncation artifact, caused by interfaces with an abrupt change in signal intensity. All pieces of wood could be found, even the smallest ones, partly because of the artifact. Dry wood has few mobile hydrogen protons and thus produces a low MRI signal. Indeed, wet or green wood contains water with mobile hydrogen protons, but water is hypointense to fat and hardly changes the T1-weighted and proton-density MR images of green wood. Fat is brighter on T1-weighted and proton-density images than on T2-weighted images. As wood is darker, the contrast between wood and fat is greater on T1-weighted and proton-density images.

T1-weighted images also have the advantages of a shorter scanning time with less motion artifact and improved signal-to-noise ratio. They are thus preferable to T2-weighted and proton-density images for identifying wood against a fat background.

In an experimental *in-vitro* model, MR (T1-weighted image) was better than CT in detecting small pieces of wood, but this remains to be confirmed in clinical practice.

Woolfson and Wesley, 1990 [239] determined that neither MRI nor CT could be used to rule out the presence of pieces of green wood (10 by 3 mm in size) in the orbit, although larger pieces of wood may be seen or excluded. Dry wood can be shown as it produces a negative or hypointense MR image, but if it remains in the tissues and absorbs water over time, it becomes more difficult to identify. Green or rehydrated wood can thus be missed by MRI.

Specht *et al.*, 1992 [77]: MRI was able to identify dry wood (golf tee with deep intracranial penetration), while CT only showed a lucent zone in the orbit. However, wood may also be missed [144].

Dalley, 1995 [233] stated that, if CT does not rule it out and a wooden foreign body is strongly suspected, MRI can give valuable details about dry wood. MRI is superior to CT in detecting dry wooden foreign bodies. Green wood, however, may be difficult to distinguish on CT and MRI.

Cartwright *et al.*, 1995 [203]: "no conclusion can be drawn on the relative value of MR and CT for imaging of organic foreign bodies."

Ho *et al.*, 1996 [166] reported that MRI did not distinguish wood from air, but the geometric form suggests the presence of wood. According to them, MRI was not better than CT (in this case). MRI and CT can both identify wood, but not confirm its absence [236, 238].

Proton-density and T2-weighted, fast spin-echo images reproduce intraorbital fat with a higher signal, which can help to identify hypointense wood, making them comparable to T1-weighted spin-echo images. Fast spin-echo requires a shorter scanning time than the standard spin-echo.

McGuckin *et al.*, 1996 [224] concluded that there is no consensus about the application of MRI and CT in acute penetrating orbitocranial injuries involving a wooden foreign body. MRI did not show an advantage over CT in this study. *In-vitro* tests revealed that spin-echo MR images of dry and green wood were always hypointense relative to fat, possibly due to the lack of mobile protons in both cases. MRI can be used to distinguish dry and green wood from fat and extracellular fluid, but cannot differentiate dry wood from air or bone fragments and likewise the dry component of green wood, the bark.

In-vitro CT is better than MRI because, with the proper window settings and optimal image contrast, it can distinguish dry and green wood from air and bone fragments. Therefore, it is preferable to start with CT because it is superior in a fresh wound in distinguishing wood from air through density measurements. In this study, MR imaging did not show an advantage over CT, but further investigation is required.

If a perforating injury by a wooden foreign body is suspected and cannot be confirmed by CT, then an MRI is certainly indicated [232], although even this can miss small pieces of dry wood [144].

Smely and Orszagh, 1999 [32]: MRI performed on the third or fourth post-traumatic day will show a low-intensity lesion with a linear configuration. If, however, performed later (day 10) an isointense signal in T1-w and a brain hypointense signal in T2-w images can be found. Adding gadolinium–DTPA, contrast enhancement in the surrounding structures or the bark zone can be clearly visible in T1-w images. MRI performed on day 64 may show a primarily hyperintense signal in T1-w; contrast application did not change the images. Thus, an intracranial wooden foreign body does not always present on MRI as a hypotense structure. Like CT imaging, MRI is influenced by the time factor.

In principle, MRI is contraindicated with ferromagnetic foreign bodies because they can move under the influence of the magnetic field, causing further damage [77, 243, 244]. Small particles, however, will not move very much, depending on their mass and shape and the properties of the magnetic field [77].

It is important to realize that both CT and MRI can miss rehydrated, wet or green wood. Thus, it is relevant to know whether the foreign body is made of green or dry wood. MRI can show better a shadow produced by dry wood, without revealing that the abnormality is indeed wood. CT examination in the acute phase can demonstrate, through density measurements, that wood is present and not air [228]. However, small pieces of wood are difficult to distinguish from air because of volume averaging [166, 229]. Occasionally, MRI can distinguish wood in a granulomatous tissue reaction during the follow-up period [228].

However, the development of these two imaging methods is by no means complete. New generations of scanners and imaging techniques may be able to identify intraorbitally and/or intracranially located wood quite readily. (Examples include high-resolution MRI, MR 3D imaging, enhanced MRI with frequency-selective fat suppression technique, etc.)

ANGIOGRAPHY

In orbitocranial penetrating injuries, damage to blood vessels is seen frequently:

Birch-Hirschfeld, 1930 [110]: 33 cases of carotid artery injury among 172 orbital injuries (6 of whom died).

De Villiers and Sevel, 1975 [1]: 5 carotid artery injuries among 10 cases of TIPI.

Kieck and De Villiers, 1984 [245]: 30% incidence of vascular injuries in a series of 109 transcranial stab wounds. Vascular spasms due to SAH can produce serious complications [245]. Of 20 transorbital stab wounds, 18 were examined by angiography and, in 11, a vascular injury was found.

Bullock and van Dellen, 1985 [194]: false aneurysms appear late in up to 10% of cases.

du Trevou and van Dellen, 1992 [48]: one in three patients with a penetrating stab wound to the brain has a vascular complication, usually treatable, and thus angiographic examination is essential. As a traumatic aneurysm can develop rapidly, angiography must be done early on. Several authors [102, 198, 247] have described traumatic aneurysms.

These data from the literature stress that a vascular injury is a definite hazard, which must be diagnosed by angiography and treated surgically. The mortality associated with hemorrhaging from traumatic aneurysms is 34% (for stab wounds to the brain in general), and a second hemorrhage is usually fatal [48]. In this series, 61 angiographic examinations were carried out. Eight carotid–cavernosus fistulae were found, 9 traumatic aneurysms and 4 carotid artery occlusions.

Several authors question the need for angiography in every case of TIPI.

Jackson *et al.*, 1971 [149] perform angiography only for deep penetrations or when the penetrating object is large. Proximity to large blood vessels or a dural sinus is also an indication [248].

van Dellen and Lipschitz, 1978 [53] do not perform angiography in acute cases where a vascular injury seems unlikely. In cases of doubt, however, angiography must be carried out and repeated.

Herring *et al.*, 1988 [54] feel that angiography is necessary whenever CT shows intracerebral, intraventricular or subarachnoid blood. Follow-up angiography is not required in every case; they consider first the severity of the injury and its proximity to large blood vessels.

Devi *et al.*, 1993 [249] wondered whether angiography was needed for simple perforating injuries through the orbital roof, with penetration of the frontal lobe, even if a hematoma is present. They called this situation 'less clear'.

I agree with De Villiers [2] that angiography is necessary and important for all transorbital injuries, because of the vascular complications which can arise. In particular, late complications highlight the responsibility of the primary treating physician [43]. An angiography should always be performed early and before surgery is undertaken [105, 144, 250].

An absolute indication for vascular examination is a penetrating body still *in situ*, which reaches as far as the large basal vessels [194, 248]. Before removing the object, angiography must be performed to evaluate the risk of a massive hemorrhage [6 case 1]. If angiography reveals an occluded carotid artery, then simply retracting the penetrating object can produce severe bleeding through the nose [163].

Controversy still exists about when and how often to perform cerebral angiography. Some authors [98, 245] feel that the examination is best performed in the second or third week after the trauma, as this will reveal a possible traumatic aneurysm. Others [48] point out that a traumatic aneurysm can arise at any moment after the trauma and can burst; a second hemorrhage is associated with a high mortality. It is better to perform angiography immediately and to treat according to the findings [55]. This seems to be the most reasonable course to take. However, even early angiography, showing a normal condition, does not exclude the possibility of a developing traumatic aneurysm. It is still possible to suffer a fatal hemorrhage late on from a previous undetected traumatic aneurysm [198].

Even if the benefit is limited, repeat angiography must be considered to reveal the late development of a traumatic aneurysm [54, 198, 245, 251]. However, even angiography performed after removal of the penetrating object does not guarantee absence of complications [53].

Patients with vasospasm or a vessel 'cut-off' aspect on angiography should have a repeat angiography [48].

12

Treatment

It goes without saying that standard treatment should always be given first; that is, stabilization of the patient's general condition, keeping open airways, treating shock, etc.

In the treatment of a patient with TIPI, other specialists should be involved in addition to the ophthalmologist and the neurosurgeon: an ENT specialist (if the sinuses are affected) and possibly a plastic surgeon (for other facial injuries) [21].

In the literature, occasionally, the ophthalmologist has carried out the initial exploration of the orbital wound [1, 24]. Only upon finding an orbital wall fracture, brain tissue or CSF was the neurosurgeon alerted. There are even descriptions of intracranial exploration through the orbit [164, 252] although modern neuroimaging has made this unnecessary. A transorbital brain injury must be considered the result of a compound, infected, comminutive impression fracture [18, 253] with all the associated consequences regarding treatment. The high risk of, for example, meningitis (25% in [211]; 21% in this series) means that surgical treatment of the compound wound is required as soon as possible [50, 164]. Late intervention only increases the risk. Miller *et al.* [24, 49, 108] found that early operation showed 33% and late operation 50% morbidity [108]. Administering antibiotics is important but not a substitute for timely surgical intervention [8]. In general, surgical treatment must be performed as soon as possible [116, 254].

Even before considering surgery, a detailed radiological examination must be performed. This examination determines the point of entry of the foreign body, the extent of bone injury, the exact location of the foreign body, which is possibly still *in situ*, and the selection of the best surgical approach. Consideration must be given to performing an angiography to rule out a traumatic aneurysm [250].

Definite indications for craniotomy are:

1. An expanding intracranial lesion;
2. Vascular injury, with hemorrhage or a traumatic aneurysm;
3. Deep-located foreign body, still *in situ*, next to important cerebral vessels;
4. Persistent liquor fistulas, pneumocephalus [98];
5. A considerable degree of splintering and embedded bone fragments.

There is no debate about these indications for surgery; however, the question remains whether every TIPI should be treated surgically. It may be that some cases can be treated conservatively: this will be dealt with below.

During craniotomy, the following aspects should be dealt with:

1. Removal of any expanding process (hematoma, abscess).
2. Removal of the foreign body or any remaining pieces. Special attention should be paid to the deepest end of the foreign body: is it intact or splintered? In the latter case, there may be pieces still *in situ.*
3. Removal of punched-in bone fragments, also from the track of the stab wound itself. Infection around bone fragments occurs 10 times more frequently than in cases without bone fragments [3].
4. Removal of extravascular blood and debriding of contused brain tissue, as necrotic tissue easily becomes infected [254].
5. Repair of vascular defects with meticulous hemostasis.
6. Excision of the dura around the defect and plastic, watertight closure. Repair of the orbital roof is generally unnecessary [255] unless there is a rise in intracranial pressure [21]. The defect fills with new fibrotic tissue, forming an effective barrier [21, 255].
7. If the paranasal sinuses or sinus frontalis are open, the mucous covering can be removed and the space filled with muscle tissue.

The choice of surgical approach to the orbitocranial transition is determined by the location of the penetration. Perforations through the orbital roof are easily accessible through a classical fronto–temporal trepanation [6, 21]. The posterior parts of the orbit, the base of the frontal lobe, the parasellar area and the temporal pole can be reached adequately. Perforations of the orbital roof primarily occur in the posterior part. The newer pteryonal approach provides access to perforations through the SOF [157], ala minor and major and the optic canal (the posterolateral part of the orbit) and the anterior temporal fossa [256]. A foreign body located in the SOF can best be approached pteryonally and extradurally [257]. With this approach only the SOF's periosteum or dura is opened, which does not communicate directly with the intracranial space, thus achieving a lower risk of surgery-induced infection [157].

Perforation through the SOF can remain extradural; thus, during intradural inspection, the situation may appear to be normal [72, 139, 157], even though it may be possible to palpate the foreign body. In cases of dura perforation, intradural inspection is indicated.

Does *every* TIPI have to be treated surgically?

Many authors recommend a formal craniotomy as the best treatment: this is called the 'open-and-see' method. Several examples include:

Dujovny *et al.* [13, 258]: the importance of formal intracranial exposure is emphasized.

Duffy and Bandari [116]: antibiotic treatment is not a substitute for surgery, infective complications can still occur. The finding of an orbital fracture is sufficient indication for an acute intervention.

Guthkelch [78]: the ideal primary treatment of a penetrating wound is still an immediate excision of all its layers.

Scarfo *et al.* [50]: surgery should be performed as soon as possible, to minimize the risk of infection.

Greene and Zabramski [259]: non-operative management unnecessarily exposes individuals with such injuries to potentially life-threatening acute hemorrhage.

Dietz [43]: da die Dura auf alle Fälle verschlossen und die Hirnverletzung versorgt werden mussen, ist ein transfrontales neurochirurgisches Vorgehen immer notwendig.

Verbiest [21]: based on our experiences, we take a more aggressive approach (exploration along the transcranial route) as chemotherapy and antibiotics do not prevent a serious intracranial complication.

Herring *et al.* [54]: we advocate surgical exploration of all such patients (transcranial stab wounds).

Nakayama *et al.* [65]: the neurosurgeon can evaluate the total situation through an open-and-see policy.

In contrast, Jackson *et al.* [149], for example, qualify the absolute viewpoint of always-surgery to some extent: "the pull-and-observe method should be reserved only for exceptional cases". The pull-and-observe method is synonymous with pull, observe and wait for complications [149], or the pull-and-see method [260], and implies retrograde removal of the foreign body via the orbit without performing a formal craniotomy, but possibly under CT monitoring [261].

The open-and-see method has a number of advantages; only then can the situation be clearly evaluated [258, 259]:

1. Remaining pieces of the foreign body, bone fragments and devitalized brain tissue can be removed, also from the stabwound itself, which could lead to a brain abscess if left *in situ* [78 case 6];
2. Check for bleeding by proximal and distal vascular monitoring [259]; only then can the foreign body be pulled out backwards;
3. Meticulous hemostasis of the cerebral wound can be performed to prevent the later development of a deep intracerebral hematoma [194];
4. Sinus defects can be closed;
5. The dura can be closed carefully.

However, surgical debridement of the wound track may increase neurological deficit. Computer-assisted surgery, providing real-time position information, may facilitate the removal of the foreign body [262].

The non-surgical pull-and-see method carries the serious risk of an immediate – or later from a traumatic aneurysm [149] – life-threatening hemorrhage. In a rapidly progressive intracerebral hematoma, even intervention by a standby neurosurgical team can be too late [259]. Retrograde removal of a foreign body from the sinus cavernosus (with angiographically confirmed carotid artery obstruction) without craniotomy, can lead to serious bleeding out of both nostrils, only controllable through carotid artery compression, enucleation of an uninjured eye and tamponade [163]. With the penetrating object still *in situ*, after an exploratory angiography, craniotomy with proximal and distal vascular control is preferred, especially with location of the foreign body in the sinus cavernosus. An object situated in the sinus cavernosus may have caused a traumatic aneurysm of the carotid artery. Simply pulling out the object may lead to heavy bleeding [6]. A foreign body must never be just pulled out [263]. It is better to expose the tip of the foreign body first via craniotomy and then to remove the foreign body under visual control backward through the entrance wound [194]. Casual removal leads to further damage; an open-and-see approach is always necessary, even for defects of the anterior fossa discovered later, and even without a CSF fistula. Exploration is essential, and the dura must be closed to prevent complications [258].

Formal trepanation to check the carotid artery proximally to and distally from the penetrating object, is required [265]. It is also possible to have an injury to the carotid artery which is initially invisible due to a normal first angiography [198]; repeat angiography somewhat later may reveal a sacculation resulting from a developing traumatic aneurysm. This aneurysm may become manifest by the development or deterioration of ophthalmoplegic symptoms. Emergency intervention is essential.

Angiography may also reveal a carotid artery thrombosis, but, even then, it makes sense to remove the foreign body only after surgical exposure of the carotid artery. In such a case, during operation, the carotid artery may appear thin, bluish and without pulsation [193].

In this series, the mortality of patients in whom the foreign body had already been removed before admission was 37%, as compared with 15% for patients admitted with the foreign body still *in situ.*

This summary of advocates of the open-and-see method still does not answer the question of whether surgery is mandatory for *every* case of TIPI. A number of authors are more flexible in their opinions: they maintain various exceptions to this rule [146].

Note: When studying this question, it became clear that not all authors make a sharp distinction between general transcranial penetrating injuries and transorbital ones [54].

For example, De Villiers [1, 2] states that for transorbital knife wounds, trepanation is not immediately required. However, the knife must be removed within 8 h under radiological monitoring in a neurosurgically equipped operating theatre. Without vascular injury, the administration of antibiotics and wait-and-see option are sufficient. Not one case of infection occurred in his series, even where pneumocephalus existed. For a transorbital injury involving a wooden object, a more aggressive approach is necessary, and immediate surgery is recommended [44].

Advocates of the wait-and-see and the pull-and-see methods refer to the transorbital prefrontal leucotomy for psychiatric patients, a method at that time leading to very few complications.

Hansen *et al.* [146] feel that the pull-and-see method can be used when the foreign body is small in diameter, cylindrical and regular in shape, via the SOF embedded in a thrombosed sinus cavernosus, in the absence fractures or bone fragments. Of course, a thorough CT study of the location and the length of the foreign body are necessary first, while CT follow-up is needed to find any granulomatous process or abscess. Nevertheless, risk exists. When, on angiography, the carotid artery appears to be practically obstructed, then retrograde removal of the foreign body can lead to a severe epistaxis [163].

If the penetrating object is small in diameter and located away from the large blood vessels, then 'blind' removal and antibiotic therapy is acceptable [248]. In unclear cases and in cases with large foreign bodies or vascular injury, surgical intervention is necessary. When angiography does not reveal vascular injury, the foreign body can be removed without trepanation, but then angiography should be repeated immediately afterwards [194]. The wait-and-see method can be considered for orbital roof perforations with limited dislocation of bone fragments and an already totally removed foreign body. For example, Solomon *et al.* [71] described four conservatively treated patients with a successful outcome. The dura may even still be intact in such fractures [155 case 1]. Kasamo *et al.* [260] applied the pull-and-see method to 7 patients with good results.

In principle, 3 treatment options exist:

1. Open-and-see, with angiographic and intracranial vascular monitoring. This method can be applied with protruding deep-lying orbitocranial foreign bodies or when the penetrating object has already been removed [12, 21, 24, 50, 65, 71 case 5, 77, 139, 149, 152, 159, 161, 193, 258 case 1, 264, 266].
2. Pull-and-see and wait for complications as a calculated risk, with angiographic controls, removal under CT monitoring and neurosurgical intervention on stand-by basis [59 cases 1–3, 66, 68, 74, 145, 160, 186, 260, 261, 267, 268].
3. Wait-and-see. With the exception of a single case [81], the foreign body had already been removed in these cases. Meticulous monitoring and antibiotic treatment are then the only activities [2, 16, 71 cases 1–4, 81, 107, 216].

Can we answer the question of which method to use in what cases based on our data? The starting point is the mortality associated with the open-

and-see versus the pull-and-see method. Mortality with the wait-and-see method is of course high (45%) partly because this group includes patients from earlier times before antibiotics and when surgical treatment was not available, as well as those patients with a severe untreatable injury.

This series shows that the mortality after surgical intervention (7%) is about the same as that after the pull-and-see method (7.5%). It is reasonable to consider this issue for modern times, choosing the data since 1977. After 1977, 66% of patients were surgically treated, while 10% were treated by the pull-and-see method. The wait-and-see method was used for 24% of patients, of whom 13 died, all of them hopeless cases. Of the surgically treated patients, two died, one because of a poor general condition. Of those treated by the pull-and-see method, only one died.

The above-mentioned data support the suggestion that, under specific conditions, conservative treatment can be considered, for example:

1. Small perforations of the orbital roof with no or only slight punching-in of the fracture, and caused by a smooth, strong object small in diameter, without hematoma or pieces of the foreign body remaining *in situ*, with normal angiographic findings.
2. Lateral or medial perforations through the SOF, with a normal angiogram (or at the most showing a thrombosis of the sinus cavernosus [146], without hematoma and/or remaining pieces of the penetrating object.

In all cases, CT follow-up is indicated.

Perforations through the medial SOF with penetration into or through the sinus cavernosus require careful handling. Angiography is always necessary. If the foreign body is still protruding from the orbit or lying deeply *in situ*, then the open-and-see method must be used. If the penetrating object is absent, then the wait-and-see option with angiographic control can be considered.

Occasionally, an author suggests craniotomy in order to extirpate the foreign body in a forward direction [66]. In general, however, the foreign body is removed backwards; craniotomy serves to prevent further injury and hemorrhage. Anterograde removal can be necessary when the object is serrated (e.g. a knife) or is a bearded arrow [55, 172, 249]. Craniotomy allows removal of the bone around the penetrating object, thus allowing easier extirpation. A foreign body must never be removed by wrenching [265]. For a serrated knife, it may be better to exert diagonal pressure in the direction of the non-serrated side of the knife [265].

Extraction of a deep-penetrating impacted sharp object, like a spear, can be achieved by using the mechanical advantage of the lever principle, thus reducing secondary damage to the minimum. The adjacent bone is used as a fulcrum; the downward force will lift the object upwards by the millimeter [30].

Surgical treatment of a brain abscess resulting from a TIPI is associated with special problems. Any remaining pieces of the penetrated object may produce renewed abscess formation [269]. The neurosurgeon must be absolute certain that all fragments of the foreign body have been removed; although occasionally patients have been described where residual parts of the foreign body remained *in situ*, apparently without causing any evident problems (tip of a pencil, [103 case 1]). Aspiration of the abscess is not sufficient; the abscess wall may contain pieces of the foreign body, which must be removed if possible. The abscess can be connected to the orbital roof by a fibrous band, which may contain pieces of the foreign body. This tract should be removed to prevent renewed abscess formation [184, 208, 270].

An absolute indication for surgical intervention is the development of a persistent CSF fistula after injury, either through the eye socket or the nose. Definitive closure of a CSF fistula can be very difficult in cases of an associated extensive comminutive fracture of the ethmoid and/or lamina cribrosa. The fistula may persist postoperatively and can even lead to a tension pneumocephalus [106].

13 Antibiotic therapy

Periorbital tissue is well vascularized and thus unlikely to become infected. The situation is different intracranially, leading to the question of whether antibiotic therapy should be administered immediately. In patients with TIPI, the issue is controversial [90]. Some authors have reservations [24]: antibiotics can mask the severity of the injury, are expensive, and carry inherent risks of allergies, idiosyncrasies and toxicity. In addition, the development of resistant Gram-negative strains may result [52, 92]. A successful prophylactic antibiotic therapy, dealing with all possible pathogenic bacteria is not available [92]. In spite of the use of broad-spectrum antibiotics, a brain abscess may still develop [21, 271]. Antibiotics cannot substitute for optimal surgical treatment with rigorous removal of all pieces of the foreign body. One cannot depend on antibiotics alone [8, 78 case 6]. Antibiotics may combat a bacterial invasion, but not if the wound contains necrotic hemorrhagic tissue or pieces of the foreign body [3].

Other authors recommend a high dose of antibiotics because of the great infection risks, even if, initially, no indication of intracranial penetration is present [12, 18, 47, 53, 54, 98, 116, 123, 152, 254, 272, 273] and even though we do not know with any degree of certainty whether it helps [5]. Some assert that infection 'usually can be prevented' [106]. In this series, we saw infections in 22% of the patients who presented after 1977, usually in the form of a brain abscess.

Staphylococcus aureus is the most common infecting agent found after TIPI [90, 108, 175, 274]. Miller *et al.* [108] noted 7 instances of *S. aureus* among 13 cultures. However, any Gram-positive or Gram-negative bacterium, present on or in the foreign body, the skin or the sinuses, can initiate infection.

Representatives of the *Bacillus* group, ubiquitous and sometimes pathogenic, such as *B. licheniformis,* can produce a brain abscess after TIPI [271, 274, 275]. Pathogens from the anaerobic *Clostridium* group (*C. perfringens* [215]) may also be found [11]. Anaerobic infections can be caused by multiple strains of anaerobic organisms, with or without aerobic specimens [276].

Occasionally, fungi are involved (*Petriellidium* (*Allescheria*) *boydii* [93]), and antibiotic therapy must be adjusted accordingly.

If antibiotic therapy is given, the coverage must be maximal; the antibiotics must have good cerebral penetration, and high bactericidal dosages must be given; this may possibly eliminate organisms before they multiply [12]. Administering a token dose is ineffective. It is advisable to follow Bard and Jarrett's advice [12]: because the stakes are so high, it is not reasonable to refrain from giving a patient at risk a massive dose of antibiotics.

The prophylactic administration of anticonvulsant medicaments for TIPI is even more controversial. Reference is made to the extensive neurological literature on the use of these drugs in cases of brain injury.

14 Complications

Complications appearing after TIPI can be classified into cerebral, orbital and vascular types.

CEREBRAL COMPLICATIONS

As early as 1905, Coqueret [20] distinguished between 'complications immédiates' and 'complications tardives'. The former included infections, brain injury in the broadest sense and carotid artery lesions with a carotid–cavernosus fistula (CCF). The latter consist primarily of brain abscesses, epilepsy, headache and changes in personality.

Duffy and Bandari [116] prefer to subdivide the late complications into late vascular and late infectious groups. Duke-Elder [8] followed this division in 1972.

Dietz [43] noted four late cases (persistent CSF fistulas, brain abscesses and recurring meningitis) in a group of 15 patients (excepting those injured by grenade splinters). Complications have also been extensively described by De Villiers [2]. Lavergne [17] stated that the cerebral complications usually involve 'late infections', but this is too limited: a variety of complications may occur at any time.

The route of cranial entry determines the pattern of complications, allowing anticipation of potential problems and treatment to be directed accordingly [6].

Early cerebral complications are:

1. Direct injury to the brain nerves, hemisphere or brainstem;
2. Infections, such as a rapidly developing meningitis, ventriculitis, brain abscess, tetanus or intracerebral gas formation;
3. Vascular injuries:
   a. Arterial lesion with an acute intracerebral, intraventricular or subdural hematoma, subarachnoid hemorrhage or the development of a traumatic aneurysm,
   b. Injury to the sinus cavernosus (or other venous sinuses) with a venous hemorrhage or thrombosis; and/or injury to the carotid artery, resulting in a traumatic aneurysm, CCF or carotid artery occlusion through thrombosis;
4. CSF fistulas;

5. Porencephalic cysts;
6. Pneumocephalus.

Late cerebral complications can be classified as:

1. Late vascular problems:
   a. CCF [1, 56, 75],
   b. Traumatic aneurysms of the carotid artery [1, 198], anterior choroidal artery [247], anterior cerebral artery [23, 102], frontopolar artery [277],
   c. occlusion of the carotid artery [1, 193];
2. Late infectious problems: brain abscesses and meningitis, apparent after a delayed period.

Direct brain injury symptoms vary according to the route of the perforating injury. The importance of a careful initial neurological examination is emphasized by case histories where only this investigation revealed the existence of a deep penetration. An example is a contralateral gaze paresis, indicating a penetration into the brainstem. Occasionally, only a temporary loss of n3 function exists, suggesting penetration up to its exit from the brainstem [200, 278].

Infections

Due to the proximity of the paranasal sinuses, infections arise more frequently with transorbital brain injuries than with brain injuries with other penetration routes [1–3]. Infections arise through:

1. Bacteria present on the penetrating object;
2. Introduction of skin bacteria;
3. Opening of the air sinuses and introduction of their bacterial flora;
4. Dragging along infected bone fragments;
5. Bacteremia and colonization of bacteria in devitalized brain tissue [92].

Infection produced by pieces of the foreign body remaining *in situ* has often been described and can arise as late as 40 or 51 years after injury [217, 279]. Organic material is especially dangerous in this respect. Let us recall Miller *et al.*'s finding [108] here: TIPI by a wooden object is associated with a higher morbidity, because of the infection rate alone. Even after introduction of the first antibiotics, they still noted, for wooden foreign bodies, an infection rate of 64%.

In this series since 1977, infection was found in 22% of cases, primarily involving brain abscesses.

Pilcher [280] demonstrated experimentally in dogs that a foreign body remaining *in situ*, reaching the ventricle system and still protruding through the skin always leads to a fatal infection. If removed within 12 h and without penetration of the ventricle system, the risk of infection is diminished.

Meningitis after TIPI can appear fulminantly, arising within 12–24 h, or after a longer time (weeks or months) [12]. In children, cases of meningitis, recurring or not, may suggest a recent or remote TIPI [189, 192].

If blood has entered the subarachnoid space because of a TIPI, then, after partial clean up of the CSF, a bacterial meningitis may become apparent [281].

In this series, 79 cases of meningitis occurred (21%), 53 of them (14%) without an associated brain abscess.

Brain abscess is a well-known and the most frequent complication after TIPI. In Miller *et al.*'s patient material [108], 48% suffered a brain abscess; in Bursick and Selker's [18], this was up to 75%. In other series, curiously enough, no mention of infection is made [260].

In this series, 19% of the patients developed a brain abscess. A brain abscess can arise in the first 3–5 weeks after the injury, but also much later, even after 40 [279] or 51 years [79]. The presence of a foreign body represents a potential danger for the development of a brain abscess. Yet, it is difficult to explain such a long symptom-free interval [3]. Several possibilities are suggested:

1. The presence of low-virulence micro-organisms;
2. Bacteremia in later years associated with local low resistance around the foreign body in the granulation tissue;
3. General lowering of resistance.

A brain abscess can be multilocular, up to 16 cavities [78 cases 4 and 5]. Occasionally, a fibrous strand is found leading to the orbital roof [171 case 3]. The additional discovery of a small scar on an eyelid may be the only indication of a previous TIPI [78 case 5]. The wall of every abscess must be thoroughly examined during operation (or autopsy) for pieces of a foreign body, occasionally found accidentally, e.g. the tip of a pencil [171 case 3, 269, 282]. If the foreign body is not found during the first operation, then, several weeks later, a recurrent brain abscess may appear. Only after removal of all remaining parts of the object can recurrence of infection be prevented [269, 270 case 1]. An ENT specialist may be called in to examine the upper nasal cavity in a case of a brain abscess. Unexpectedly, the remains of a pencil may be sometimes found high up in the nose, even though the patient does not know how it got there [179].

A piece of wood lying in the SOF can lead to a recurrent brain abscess in the temporal lobe [208].

Ventriculitis

The perforating agent can reach the ventricle system directly and produce a fulminant ventriculitis in a child, which may be fatal within 32 h [49].

Pneumocephalus [59, 93, 106, 283, 284]

A transorbital injury through the lamina papyracea, ethmoid sinus and lamina cribrosa or directly through a pneumatized part of the orbital roof can easily produce a pneumocephalus. As already detailed in the chapter on anatomy, the dura is securely fixed to the bone in the region of the anterior cranial fossa and thus does not move readily. In addition, the dura is thin in that area, tears easily and heals poorly. In the bone–dura opening thus produced, a CSF fistula can develop or a prolapse of arachnoid, brain tissue or sinus mucosa [211]. When blowing the nose or sneezing, air can be forced intracranially and then be sealed in by a valve mechanism. Alternatively, CSF may be simply replaced by air. The air can essentially reside in epidural, subdural, or subarachnoid spaces, or intracerebrally or intraventricularly [285]. On radiological examinations, intracerebrally trapped air can appear pear-shaped with a tract to the site of perforation [211].

Twenty-five per cent of pneumocephalus arises within the first week and 75% within the first 3 months [211]. Only repeated radiological examinations may reveal a pneumocephalus.

Pneumocephalus may be the first and only indication of a transorbital injury [211, 285].

Intracranially trapped air may lead to clinical signs or may cause aspecific complaints, such as headaches and nuchal rigidity. Sometimes, upon head movements, a splashing sound is heard. Even without symptoms, nevertheless, an open connection exists between the intracranial contents and the outside environment, with the associated risk of a serious infection.

The valve mechanism can produce a tension-pneumocephalus, with raised ICP due to the mass effect of the air, leading to neurological deterioration [11, 106]. Treatment with only a drain leads to the risk of more air being sucked in.

Pneumocephalus occurred in 17 patients in this series, of whom two had an aerocele and one a tension-pneumocephalus.

CSF leakage

This can occur temporarily through an eyelid wound or a conjunctiva injury. Occasionally, a leak into the eye socket may occur with severe chemosis and eyelid edema [71]. Epiphora can be due to a CSF leak [71]. CSF fistulas through the nose are well known and do not need to be discussed here. Persistent CSF loss is unusual [6], as a fresh dura lesion with CSF leakage closes spontaneously in 80% of patients within 72 h [71]. Persistent CSF loss must be treated, as 25% of dura lesions are associated with meningitis [106, 211].

Porencephalia

Porencephalic cysts can arise when the perforating object reaches the ventricle system through a fracture in the orbital roof [286]. If this is accompanied by a raised ICP (for example, due to an obstructive hydrocephalus), the porencephalic cyst may gradually extend into the orbit by pulsation and erosion. This can lead to a pulsating exophthalmus [286].

ORBITAL COMPLICATIONS

We shall consider only complications of importance to the neurosurgeon. Ocular injuries are not included here. The eyeball is usually spared in low-velocity TIPI involving pointed thin objects, which are more likely to displace the eyeball than traumatize it.

In our material, the eyeball was intact in 74% of patients (in 12% there was a defect of the eyeball; in 14% the condition of the eyeball was not mentioned). Sclera perforation is associated with a poor prognosis for vision: only 55% of these patients reported some return of vision [128].

Optical nerve damage

Birch-Hirschfeld [110] found 125 (73%) optical nerve injuries among 172 stab wounds of the orbit (traversing or not). It is characteristic not only to suffer loss of vision but also to develop a relative afferent pupil reflex defect, the well-known Marcus–Gunn pupil. An isolated loss of the afferent pupil reflex does not lead to a difference in pupil diameter. However, with the uninjured eye closed, the pupil on the injured side dilates, which can be misleading ('epidural hematoma') if the consensual reaction is not tested.

Post-traumatic amaurosis indicates direct n2 injury and/or vascular injury of the ophthalmic artery or central retinal artery with retinal ischemia and a pale edematous fundus [157]. The ophthalmic artery meets the n2 in the anterior third of the nerve's orbital course and is then called the central retinal artery. Injury to this anterior one third of the n2 causes obstruction of the central retinal artery and thus retinal ischemia. Injury posterior to this point is initially associated with a normal fundus, but later optical nerve atrophy develops.

Acute blindness after orbital penetration has an unfavorable prognosis for vision, but sometimes, after removing the foreign body, vision can be restored [196, 203], even months later [186], except when n2 atrophy has occurred. Thus, acute total blindness is not necessarily permanent unless CT reveals a transection of the optical nerve. Late removal of wooden foreign bodies from the orbit can lead to dramatic improvements also in eye motility disturbances, even 1 year after the accident [230, 287, 288].

Sebag *et al.* [187] stated that vision is rarely spared in TIPI. In our material, an n2 injury occurred in 34% of the surviving patients, in 11% without damage to the oculomotor nerves (n3, n4, and n6). The n2 and the ophthalmic artery run close together in the posterior orbit and thus are often simultaneously injured here [273].

In the first phase after TIPI, it is difficult to give a prognosis regarding vision. The examination is often difficult to perform, and vision may spontaneously return, even in cases of penetration involving a long wooden object [210]. Occasionally, a prognosis can be made only after 4–6 weeks [18]. Visually evoked potentials may give an indication of the vision prognosis.

Injury to the oculomotor nerve (n3), trochlear nerve (n4), abducens nerve (n6) and the first trigeminal nerve branch (n5,1)

Penetration of the orbital wall often occurs through the SOF (30% in our series), where these nerves lie in close proximity. n3 and n6, in particular, are commonly injured as they lie medially, in the wider portion of the SOF. n4 is situated more laterally in the SOF and somewhat removed from the usual penetration route [6]. n4 injury can occur while the n2 remains intact.

Damage to this group of nerves can also occur immediately behind the SOF in the lateral wall of the sinus cavernosus, leading to an SOF syndrome. The n3 has a short intraorbital course before dividing into upper and lower branches. This short course is closely associated with the optic nerve [150]. A combined injury is not unusual here [8, 150].

It is often difficult to judge the degree of injury to the oculomotor nerves in the initial phase and whether the loss is permanent.

Injury to the orbital wall bordering on the paranasal sinuses, such as the lamina papyracea, can lead to orbital emphysema (primarily with fractures of the medial orbital wall), cellulitis, abscess formation, CSF fistulas, pneumocephalus and meningitis. Occasionally, ophthalmologic examination of the orbit may reveal necrotic brain tissue; in earlier days, this was sometimes the first indication of a TIPI. With the current imaging technology, this is no longer an issue.

Eye pulsations, synchronous with the heart rate, with or without exophthalmus, may be of diagnostic significance in cases of: traumatic orbital arteriovenous fistula [289], carotid–cavernosus fistula, or an extensive orbital roof defect with a potential prolapse of brain tissue [71 case 4, 91, 187 case 3]. These pulsations may be the only symptom of a perforating injury. A pulsating exophthalmos can also be due to a giant traumatic aneurysm of the anterior cerebral artery, as a result of a perforating injury of the orbital roof [102]. Furthermore, it can also arise after an orbital roof defect in association with a pre-existing subclinical hydrocephalus [255] or raised intracranial pressure due to other causes, such as a space-occupying lesion in the posterior fossa [91] and hydrocephalus developing after an orbital roof defect [24 case 3]. A large orbital roof defect, caused by neurosurgical intervention, does not lead by itself to a pulsating exophthalmus, because of the subsequent formation of a sturdy connective tissue plate, effectively replacing the orbital roof [255]. A porencephalic cyst developing after a TIPI into the ventricle can, if an obstructive hydrocephalus develops later, extend into the orbit via the old orbital fracture by its pulsating force. The old fracture becomes widened and finally an exophthalmus, pulsating or not, can arise as the result of an intraorbital CSF cyst [286]. The connection between the intraorbital cyst and the intracerebral porencephalic cyst can be demonstrated by MRI [286]. Incidentally, intraorbital CSF cysts have also been reported after orbital roof fractures by other causes not considered here.

It can be difficult to distinguish an intraorbital CSF cyst from a traumatic implantation cyst of the conjunctiva [290]. Implantation cysts of the conjunctiva are rare, representing only 10% of intraorbital epidermoid and dermoid cysts [290]. For diagnostic identification, transorbital cyst puncture, RISA, metrizamide cysternography or CT imaging can be used, but MRI is currently the best choice [286].

Orbital liquorrhea or orbitorrhea has been described occasionally after TIPI [174, 195, 257]. Temporary CSF loss, usually in the form of bloody fluid or 'serosanguineous fluid', sometimes mixed with brain tissue, can flow from the eyelid or conjunctiva wound.

In this series, this occurred 21 times, occasionally as copious leakage. A CSF leak in the orbit can be shown by Tc-99m DTPA cisternography (Figure 31) [291]. Severe eyelid edema and/or epiphora can be due to CSF

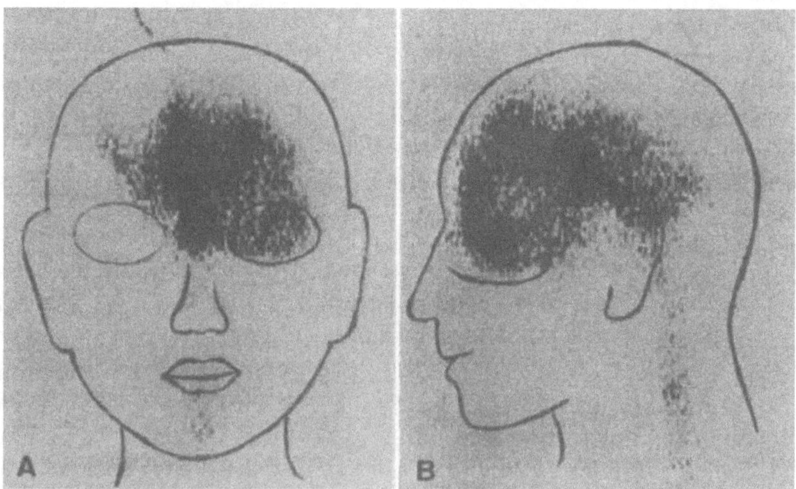

Figure 31 CSF leak in the orbit, as shown by Tc-99m DTPA cisternography

leakage in the orbit [71]. Occasionally, the CSF leakage into the eye socket persists; standard conservative treatment measures, such as raising the head and reducing CSF pressure, may be ineffective [195]. These cases must be treated surgically, especially if the foreign body is still *in situ* [174].

VASCULAR COMPLICATIONS

These complications include:

1. Direct or indirect (e.g. due to bone fragments) injury of a cerebral blood vessel with acute bleeding;
2. Development of a traumatic aneurysm;
3. Injury to the sinus cavernosus;
4. Carotid artery injury, usually involving the fixed intracavernous portion, leading to the development of a carotid–cavernosus fistula, carotid thrombosis [88], traumatic aneurysm or even transection of the vessel;
5. Vascular spasms.

According to Kieck and De Villiers, transorbital stab wounds are associated with a high incidence of vascular injury at the base of the brain [245].

Among 18 transorbital stab wounds, examined angiographically between 2 and 3 weeks after injury, they found 11 patients with a vascular injury:

- 4 carotid–cavernosus fistulas, developing 48–72 h after the injury;
- 3 aneurysms;
- 1 carotid artery occlusion, 1 transection;
- 2 delayed vascular spasms, caused by the presence of blood in the CSF.

Patients with *transcranial* stabwounds, on angiographic examination, show vascular abnormalities in 30% [245]. For *transorbital* injuries, the percentage appears to be higher. In 1975, De Villiers found 50% carotid artery lesions among 10 transorbital stab injuries. Birch-Hirschfeld [110] noted 33 carotid artery lesions with a pulsating exophthalmus among 172 orbital stab wounds (19%); 6 of the 33 died.

We found, in this series, 31 vascular injuries (8.5%):

- 14 carotid–cavernosus fistulas;
- 12 traumatic aneurysms;
- 5 carotid artery occlusions.

Angiography was performed 61 times, establishing vascular injury in 21 cases (34%).

Clearly, angiography is an essential tool in the further examination of TIPI [250].

Direct damage to the large brain arteries leads to a rapidly expanding intracerebral hematoma or SAH, and surgical intervention is usually of little of no help.

The localization of a traumatic aneurysm [198, 247] is of course related to the path of the penetrating object [102]. (See Addendum 1 below.) This vascular injury can arise from direct penetration, shearing forces or broken-off sharp bone fragments. The injury to the vascular wall may be incomplete, with gradual development of an aneurysm, or complete, with the development of a hematoma and subsequent organization and hemodynamic cavitation. Also, the hematoma itself may expand and burst, leading to further damage [198]. This type of hemorrhage can arise within hours of the injury [245]. Sudden death can also occur later (after several weeks) due to bleeding from a traumatic aneurysm of e.g. the anterior choroidal artery [247].

Angiographically, a traumatic aneurysm is characterized by an irregular contour and the absence of a neck [251], requiring a trapping operation instead of clipping it. In chronic cases, a thick calcified wall may be found.

Traumatic aneurysms are not static; they can alter rapidly and develop unexpectedly [48, 234] and thus follow an unpredictable clinical course [251]. They can arise on the day of injury [247], even within hours [250], or develop very slowly. They are rarely caused by wooden foreign bodies [234]. Thus, the initial angiographic examination may appear normal, even without vascular spasms [198, 251].

A traumatic aneurysm can expand, shrink, or even disappear entirely due to thrombosis. Late-appearing traumatic aneurysms can be expected in 10% of all brain injuries in which the skull has been penetrated [194].

The incidence of SAH is high (71% [245]), and the prognosis of a patient with a traumatic aneurysm involving the circle of Willis and its branches is poor. The demonstration of a traumatic aneurysm demands emergency surgery [198, 245].

In this series, I found 12 traumatic aneurysms; 6 of these patients died. The true incidence must be higher as angiographic examination was introduced only in later years.

Perforation of the sinus cavernosus

Injury to the sinus cavernosus occurs with transorbital perforations through the medial part of the SOF. Perforation of the wall of the sinus by itself can be dangerous [76]. An intermittently leaking thrombus may form in the tear in the wall, leading to recurrent episodes of meningeal irritation through SAH. The thrombus can also suddenly dislodge (described after PEG and LP), resulting in massive hemorrhage. An obstructing thrombus may develop in the sinus. Combinations of carotid artery injury with fistula formation and perforation of the dilated posterior part of the sinus (most likely also perforated by the foreign body) do exist and can lead to a late fatal bleeding [292].

A pulsating exophthalmus arising after a TIPI, is not necessarily caused by a CCF, and, conversely, a CCF is not always associated with a pulsating exophthalmus [293]. However, if a pulsating exophthalmus develops soon after a TIPI, then the carotid artery is most likely injured behind the SOF in the sinus cavernosus.

De Villiers [54] noted, quite rightly, that it is actually favourable if the injury to the carotid artery as a result of TIPI occurs in the intracavernous fixed part of the internal carotid artery, as a life-threatening intracranial hemorrhage does not necessarily occur immediately.

In this series, we found 5 cases of carotid artery occlusion (one patient died), while 14 suffered a CCF (4 died).

Carotid artery injury can also arise after a perforating injury, fracturing the sphenoid [198]. A thrombosis or a traumatic aneurysm of the internal carotid artery can result or a hematoma around the artery may develop, leading to a false aneurysm with rupture. This rupture can occur through the fracture with exsanguination through the nasopharynx [198, 234]. A CCF can develop contralaterally if the penetrating injury has crossed the midline via the ethmoid [245] (see Addendum 2 below).

Repeated neurological examination with new findings, such as deterioration of n6 function, not previously noted, may be an early sign of a developing traumatic cavernous aneurysm [198] or CCF [199].

Occasionally, severe vascular spasms were recorded after TIPI, caused by hemorrhagic CSF (or possibly direct vascular injury) [245, 246]. These vascular spasms can appear in the area supplied by both anterior cerebral arteries, resulting in bilateral permanent frontal lobe damage. This is a serious complication leading to severe behavioral disturbances [245, 246].

Addendum 1.

A characteristic case was published by de Grood [23]: A 5-year-old girl was admitted (in 1965) after being stabbed with a pointed pencil in the medial canthus of the left eye. Local inspection only showed a minor injury with some bleeding. For the first 12 h after the accident, the child showed no clinical symptoms, but then high fever and nuchal rigidity developed. Lumbar puncture demonstrated hemorrhagic CSF, but also pleiocytosis (7000/3 cells). Meningitis was diagnosed and the child treated accordingly. However, high temperatures persisted and the CSF remained hemorrhagic.

It was only after 3 months that the fevers subsided and the child improved. To exclude a brain abscess, bilateral angiography was performed, and a contralateral aneurysm of the right a. cerebri anterior, near the a. communicans anterior was demonstrated. The location of the aneurysm was in line with the direction of the path of penetration.

Addendum 2.
Most likely, the first description of a contralateral carotid artery injury with the development of a CCF was the famous observation in 1855 by Auguste Nelaton (1807–1873) [cited in 7, 20 obs. 5]. The patient was a 21-year-old man, injured by an umbrella in his *left* eye. He suffered a nosebleed. Several days later, he developed a protrusion of the *right* eye with total ophthalmoplegia and a right-sided pulse-synchrone bruit. One month after the accident, the patient was examined by Nelaton who diagnosed a midline crossing injury of the contralateral sinus cavernosus, with the development of a CCF. After several serious epistaxis episodes, the patient finally died after 3.5 months. Suppey conducted an autopsy and confirmed Nelaton's brilliant diagnosis. He found a comminutive fracture of the orbital apex on the left side, extending into the sphenoid. A bone fragment had practically severed the carotid artery. Nelaton was later able to reproduce this injury on a cadaver; this preparation is reputedly still present in the Musée Dupuytren, Paris, France.

15
Aggression

In this series, 84 TIPI injuries were the result of aggressive behavior; 89% of the cases were caused by men and 11% by women. The Re/Le localisation was indicated in 78 cases. The left orbit was injured in 70.5% and the right in 29.5% (Figure 32). Thus, indeed, a right-handed attacker is more likely to hit the left side of the opponent's face or orbit, as is repeatedly suggested in literature [53, 121, 294, 295].

The weapon of aggression was most often a knife (33%) or an umbrella (33%). The mortality after injury with an umbrella was four times greater than with a knife (Figure 33). Thus, an umbrella causes more intracranial

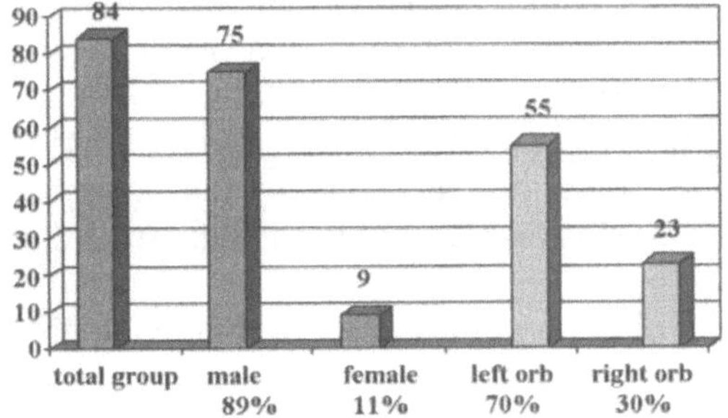

Figure 32 Aggression group: gender and right/left distribution

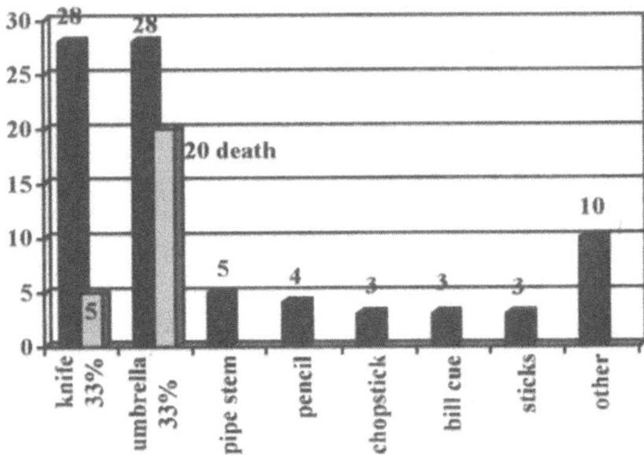

Figure 33 Objects used during aggression

damage than a knife, which can sometimes stab deeply transorbitally and intracranially without clinical evidence of neurological injury.

It is curious that umbrella injuries involve the left orbit nearly four times as often, whereas, with knives, the left is involved only twice as often as the right orbit (Figure 34). The total mortality associated with TIPI through aggression was 44%.

For comparison a few data from the literature are presented:

- 83% of assault-related penetrating ocular injuries are found in men, with the left eye being injured more often (53.8% [296]).
- Two thirds of stab wounds to the head are located on the left side, and 19% enter the orbit [48].
- De Villiers [2] noted that orbital stab wounds are as often on the left as on the right, with a mortality of 30%, but his number of patients was limited to 10 cases.

In this context, Kitahara *et al.*'s opinion is interesting [297]: they found that TIPI due to aggression was more likely to occur through the posterior part of the orbital roof, with a more median and horizontal direction. This produces more brain injury compared with a fall or an accidental TIPI, which are oriented more upwards and sagittally and thus more likely injure the frontal lobe, leading to lower morbidity and mortality (Figure 35). Indeed, this series shows that mortality in the aggression-related group (44%) was almost twice as high as that in the fall group (24%) or accidental TIPI group (22%).

In this series, the direction of the path of the penetrating object was:

- For fall trauma: 55% penetrated through the orbital roof, always leading to frontal lobe injury; 20% penetrated through the SOF;

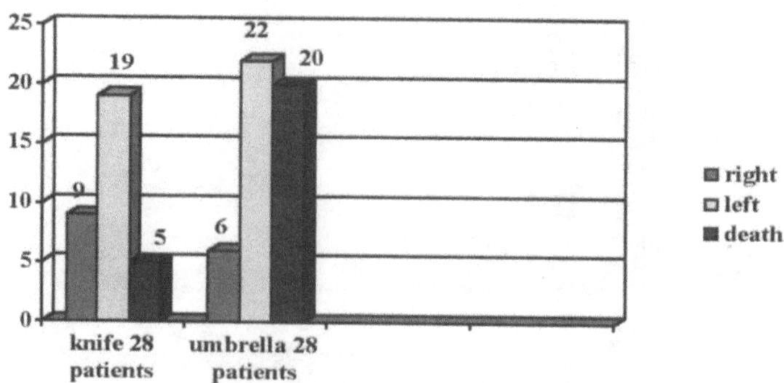

Figure 34 Umbrellas penetrate the left orbit more often, as compared with knives

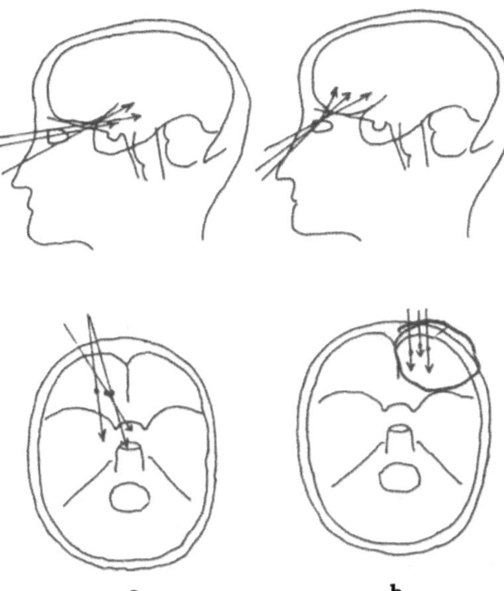

Figure 35 The site and direction of TIPI, differentiated by the cause of the injury, according to Kitahara *et al.* [297]. (a) TIPI caused by fighting. (b) TIPI caused by fall or accident

- For accident: 49% through the orbital roof, 30% through the SOF;
- For aggression: 27% through the orbital roof and 19% through the SOF.

Thus, TIPI by aggression follows the path through the orbital roof less often (1 : 2), compared with accidental and fall TIPI; other penetration routes are more frequent, resulting in more serious injury.

16
Accident

The group of patients suffering a TIPI because of an accident numbered 114. Their gender was recorded in 106 cases: 87% were male and 13% female (Figure 36). The age curve reveals that the risk of an accidental TIPI is largest between the ages of 6 and 12 years (Figure 37). In this group, the right orbit (56%) was involved more often than the left (44%). The penetrating object was most likely some sort of stick or metal rod, probably carried mainly in the right hand (Figure 38). The mortality in this group was 22%, and the morbidity of the survivors was 16%. Regarding the path taken, 49% penetrated through the orbital roof and 30% through the SOF.

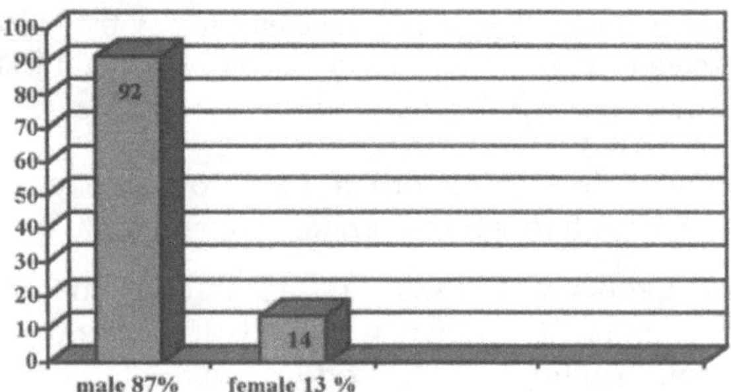

Figure 36 Gender distribution of accidental TIPI

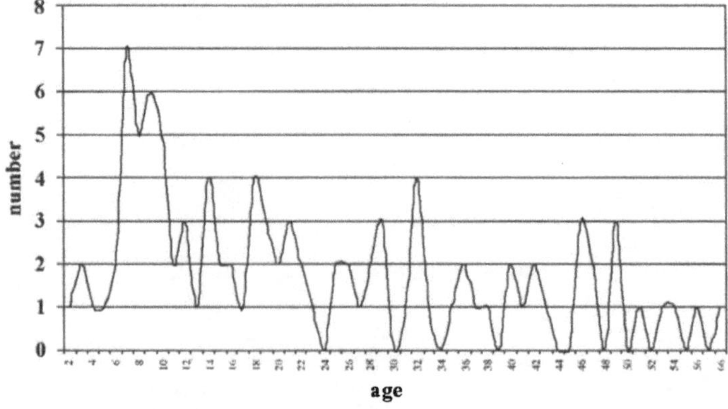

Figure 37 Age distribution of accidental TIPI

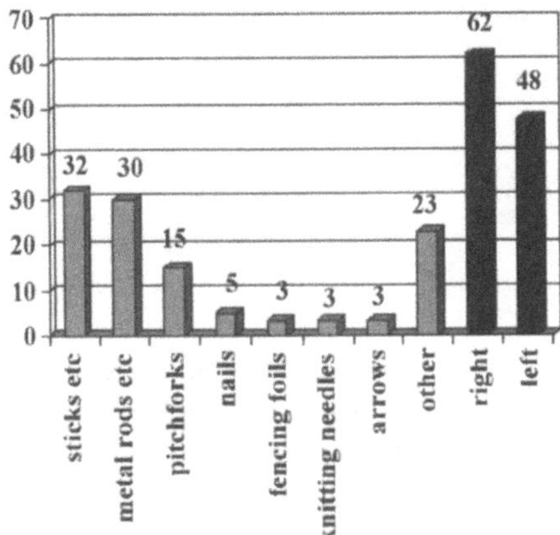

Figure 38 Objects and right/left distribution in accidental TIPI; 114 patients

17
Fall injuries

In this series, of 347 TIPI patients, a fall was the cause of injury in 130 (38%) (Figure 16). The term 'fall injury' is used in a broad sense here, every patient who suffered an orbital traversing injury as the result of a fall is included; supplemented by a few unusual cases with an extraorbital course of penetration.

The most typical accident scenario involves a young child falling down while holding a pencil, slate-pencil, ballpoint pen, etc. (Figure 39). Children fall in a different way compared with adults, i.e. more passively. They hold onto the object and do not show a tendency to break the fall by stretching out an arm. Therefore, an object held in the hand can penetrate the eye socket. A pencil is thus potentially a lethal object [18, 172]. The object can also penetrate the nose, the cheek, the pharynx or the thin temporal bone.

In this series of patients, 80% were younger than 12 years. Bursick and Selker [202] noted in their material of probable fall injuries that 82% were under 10 years of age. Adults (over 20 years old) are far less likely to suffer a TIPI due to a fall: only 15% (Figure 40).

The start of the age curve (1–16 years) of all TIPI injuries (347 cases) concerns primarily fall injuries (Figure 41a,b).

We found injuries to males in 72%, to females in only 28%. The right orbit was involved twice as often as the left (Figure 42). This reflects the right-handed dominance in the general population and is the opposite of aggressive injuries, where the left orbit is affected more often.

As expected, knives and umbrellas figure less often in fall injuries. The penetrating object is most often a stick, pen or metal rod, with various characteristics (Figure 43). Pens, pencils and ballpoint pens causing TIPI, will be dealt with in more detail later.

A fall trauma is often generalized as a 'pencil injury' or 'pencil puncture injury' [202]. Although any pointed thin object could be involved in a fall injury, Kosaki *et al.* [298] proposed the collective term 'pencil injury'. This term was first used, not by Pitner in 1966 [299] as Kosaki states, but by Bickerstaff in 1964 [300], who described cases of carotid artery thrombosis due to a penetrating oropharyngeal injury, as a result of a fall of a child having an object in his mouth.

We report several unusual penetrations, not through the orbit, caused by a fall, without being exhaustive.

(a)

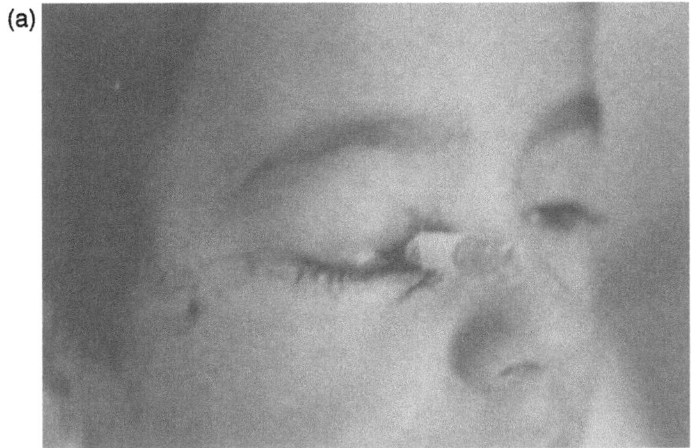

(b)

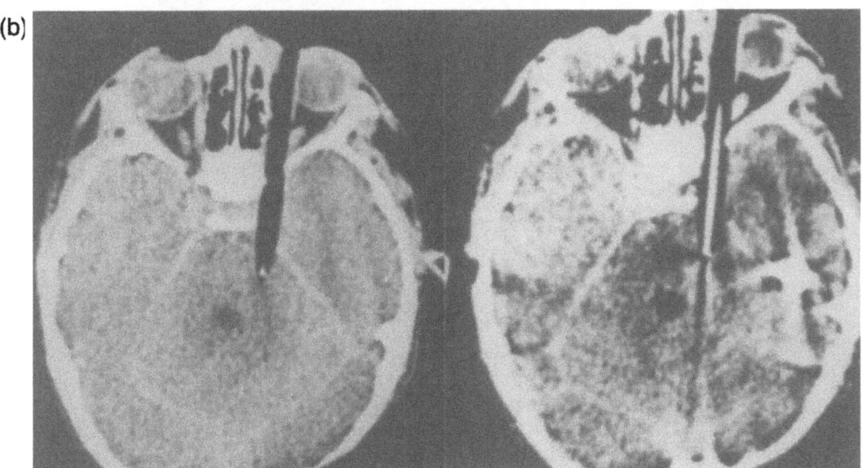

Figure 39 (a) Fall TIPI with a deep penetrating pencil. (b) CT showing the deep penetrating pencil.

Of course, the injury can be limited to the orbita [151 case 2, 203, 209, 231, 240, 287]. Occasionally, an author describes a trauma which appeared to be restricted to the orbit, but, from the length of the penetrating object (more than 5 cm), it can be deduced that symptom-free intracranial penetration must have occurred.

In children, a fall trauma can perforate the thin temporal bone [172 2×, 238, 270, 301, 302], usually resulting in an acute subdural hematoma or a temporal brain abscess.

Fall injuries with penetration through the orbital floor, extending to the sinus maxillaris, have been described [7 case 12, 99, 166, 168]. The object

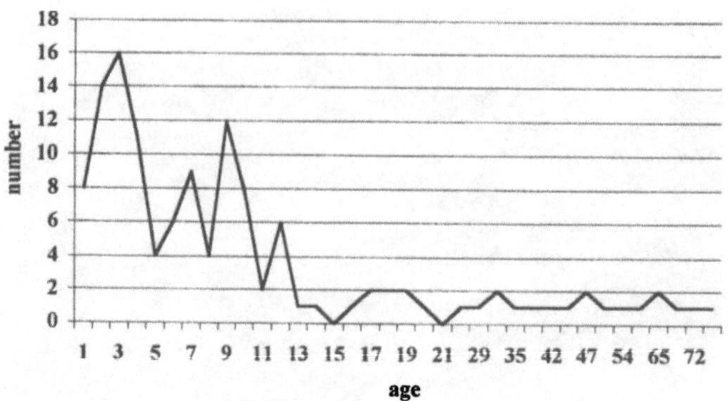

Figure 40 Age distribution of fall TIPI; 128 patients

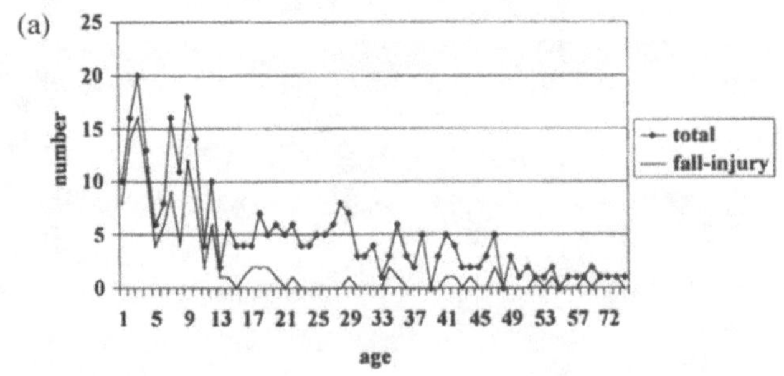

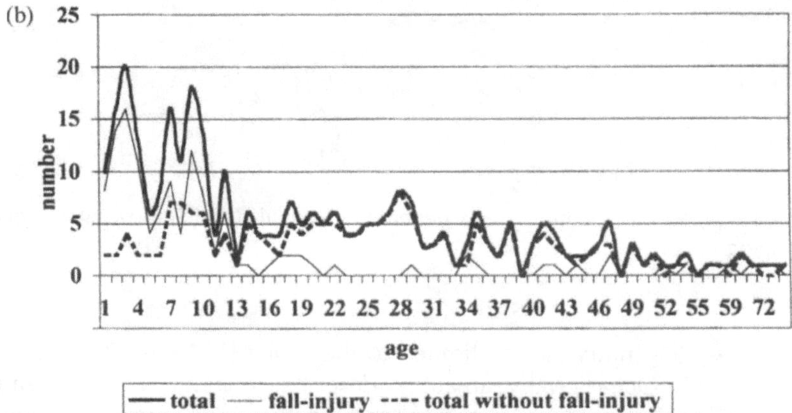

Figure 41 (a) Overall age curve compared with the fall-injury age curve. (b) The first part of the overall age curve consists mainly of fall-injury cases.

can even penetrate under the base of the skull and be palpable under the skin at C1, without causing significant injury [168]. Penetration into the sinus maxillaris is generally harmless, with complete recovery after removal of the foreign body. The fall injury object can also penetrate the cheek,

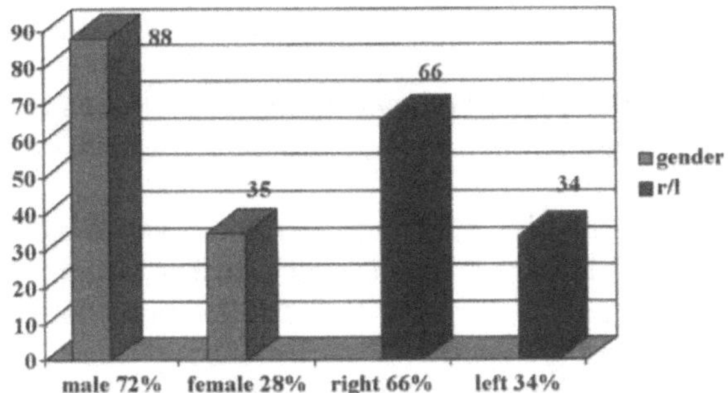

Figure 42 Gender (123 patients) and right/left (100 patients) distributions in TIPI cases caused by a fall

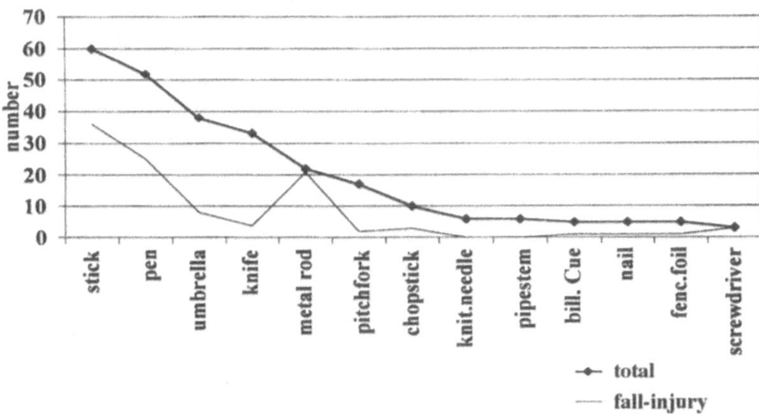

Figure 43 Object and fall-injury

then through the orbit into the temporal lobe or via the sinus maxillaris into the oropharynx [40, 303].

Fall injuries penetrating the mouth are more serious. After a few publications by previous authors, Bickerstaff [300] in 1964 associated apparently inexplicable hemiplegia in children with an oropharyngeal para-tonsillar blunt injury due to falling with an object in the mouth, leading to injury to and thrombosis of the carotid artery and thrombus propagation to the circle of Willis. He coined the term 'pencil injury' for this intraoral trauma.

In addition, retropharyngeal emphysema, abscesses, mediastinitis or pneumomediastinum can arise.

In 1964, Markham *et al.* [304] published a case of oral penetration with intracranial extension through the base of the skull.

In 1966, Pitner [299] reviewed 10 cases and added 2 patients of his own. Their ages ranged from 1 to 18 years; 8 boys and 4 girls. Nine patients fell down while carrying the penetrating object in their mouths. Two patients fell on a protruding object; one fall involved an intraoral thrust to the tonsillar area with a toy sabre.

In 1984, Hengerer *et al.* [305] were able to review 15 cases and they added one case of their own. Five deaths occurred; only 3 patients recovered.

In 1989, Mains and Nagle [31] described a five-and-a-half-year-old boy who fell, forcing the blunt end of a dowel into his mouth. Carotid artery occlusion developed with a cerebral infarct. The boy made a reasonable recovery over a period of 1 year.

This type of injury is rarely seen among adults and then has an entirely different pathogenesis – no fall injury but e.g. a punch to the jaw which dislocates false teeth.

Symptoms sometimes appear directly afterwards but usually there is a symptom-free interval of 3–48 h [305]. With a concomitant cerebral injury, this symptom-free interval can be confused with the lucid interval associated with an epidural hematoma.

The mortality associated with this specific injury is high; 1 out of 3 patients dies.

The prognosis is determined by thrombus propagation in the carotid artery to the circle of Willis. Kosaki *et al.* [298] described 12 cases in 1992. These mostly involved children who fell with a pointed object in their mouths. Carotid artery thrombosis can lead within 48 h to severe neurological symptoms. In Japan, a chopstick is often the agent of injury.

Smyth *et al.* [306] in 1996 reported four cases: 3 fall injuries and 1 forward acceleration with a screwdriver in the mouth. These were also apparently innocuous injuries, which could easily be missed. Occult perforation is possible.

In summary, a fall injury involving the mouth takes place in circumstances comparable to those of a TIPI fall injury.

The fall injury can also penetrate through the nose. In 1992, Fallon *et al.* [181] reviewed 6 cases from the literature and added 1 case of his own. However, they were not all fall injuries [64, 79, 180]: the case described by Key *et al.* [307] penetrated through the mouth and the one reported by Davis [176] is unclear. Here, too, children 2–17 years old were involved; initial examination of their injuries did not suggest an intracranial injury caused by penetration via the nose or a foreign body remaining *in situ* [175, 176, 178, 179, 269].

As an aside, a curious case is described by Keningsberg *et al.* [308] involving a pencil penetrating through the perineum of a 3-year-old boy.

SOME PATHOGENETIC CONSIDERATIONS IN FALL INJURIES

The penetrating object does not have its own kinetic energy. Therefore, penetration stops as soon as the force causing the penetration ceases.

A fall approximately in the sagittal plane upon the orbital region will always be interrupted by the bony surroundings of the orbit, namely the base of the nose, the rim of the eye-socket and the zygoma. At that point the fall stops. Therefore, the object, due to its lack of kinetic energy, will not penetrate further. The other end of the object will protrude from the eye socket (Figure 39).

Two comments must be made here:

1. If the penetrating object breaks, the broken-off piece can remain deep in the orbit and cranium, and thus no protrusion from the socket is present [59 case 2].
2. If the fall is more upon the lateral orbital lower rim, the object can penetrate all the way to the edge of the orbit, but not deeper. Its end may not be visible, but can be palpated just under the edge of the orbit [140, 148]. *Vice versa,* if the entire penetrating object is located deep orbitointracranially, a fall cannot be the cause; aggression or attempted suicide must be suspected [309]. In these cases, the object must have been pushed deep into the orbit or it must have had kinetic energy of its own, e.g. after firing by string shooting. These considerations may be of importance in forensic TIPI cases.

In adults (over 20 years old), fall injuries do occur (15%) but the course is usually different from that in children. In this series, in adults, the cause was never a fall while holding a small thin object, such as a pencil or a ballpoint pen, in the hand, but as a rule concerned a fall upon a fixed protruding object. There were 20 cases of fall injuries involving patients older than 20 years:

- 9 fell into a bush or onto a stick;
- 5 fell upon an umbrella or one of its spokes;
- 5 fell on various objects (doorknob, windowpane, agricultural machine, a key protruding from a lock [26], motorbike stand, and, in one case, the object was unknown).

An unusual case is described in which eye socket penetration occurred in a child holding a pencil, whose arm was knocked [268].

The mortality associated with fall injuries in this series was 24%. In 55%, penetration was through the orbital roof with a concomitant injury of the frontal lobe. Penetration via the SOF was seen in 20% (in 11 cases passage through the SOF was judged most likely).

De Villiers [2] stated that traversing fall injuries almost always involved penetration of the orbital roof with concomitant injury of the frontal lobe. This is the result of the protective reaction of throwing the head backwards as an object approaches the eyes and possibly the head being forced backward during the fall.

A fall onto a pencil can produce severe injury in a child; this can quickly be fatal (19 h) due to ventricular hemorrhage [116 case 5]. On the other hand, the point of a pencil can easily reach the posterior fossa through the SOF, without causing neurological and/or vascular injury along its path, except in the eye socket itself, with loss of n2, n3, n4, n6 and first trigeminal branch function [261].

18

TIPI caused by umbrellas

The umbrella is an important etiological agent causing TIPI.

In this series, 40 patients had been injured by an umbrella (11%). Even with umbrella injuries, the external visible lesion may be minor, as in a pencil fall injury, although frequently intracranially major destruction can occur [310 case 3, 311].

Men are primarily affected (87%). The distribution of this injury according to age categories is, as expected, very different from the overall age curve of TIPI; injuries caused by an umbrella appear in older age groups (Figure 44).

This injury is usually caused by aggression (72% of cases) and in only 18% by a fall. The overall mortality of 56% in TIPI cases caused by umbrellas confirms this apparently harmless utensil as a lethal weapon.

Before 1914, the mortality was higher (87.5%), mostly due to intracranial infections. After 1914, the mortality dropped to 35%; the most common causes of death since 1914 were hemorrhage (62%) and direct brain injury, primarily to the hypothalamus. For the whole series, of the survivors (44%), 41% suffered permanent damage (blindness, hemiparesis).

Of all the TIPI patients who died after 1977, the agent responsible was an umbrella in 50%.

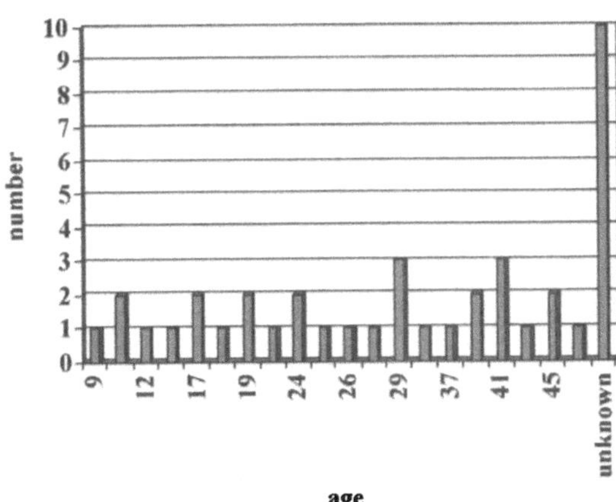

Figure 44 Age distribution of patients with a TIPI caused by an umbrella

Thus, an umbrella with ferrule is a formidable stabbing weapon for attack or self-defence. Penetration through the eye socket can easily be fatal due to intracranial infection, hemorrhage or direct brain injury, particularly of the hypothalamus.

19

TIPI caused by pencils, slate pencils and ballpoint pens

The earliest description of such an injury was produced by Hewitt [312] in 1848 (Figure 45).

In 1965 Albert *et al.* [161] reported that "transorbital pencil injuries appear to form a distinct subgroup" of TIPI, because:

- An accidental fall on a pencil occurs frequently;
- Young children are involved;
- The eyeball remains intact;
- Penetration of the roof of the orbit occurs;
- Frontal lobe abscesses frequently occur;
- There is high mortality.

In 1981, Bursick and Selker [202] devoted an entire article to 'pencil puncture injury' based on 22 case histories. A summary of their data can be found in Chapter 23.

From Miller *et al.*'s publication of 1977 [108], we selected 19 patients with a pencil puncture injury from the total group of 42 patients.

This subgroup showed the following characteristics:

- Age: 2–24 years, 14 under 10 years old (74%);
- Gender: 13 male (68%), 6 female;
- Orbit: 14 right (74%), 5 left;
- Penetration of orbital roof: 12 (63%), only 1 through the SOF;
- Penetration of upper eyelid: 11 (58%);
- Intracranial infection: 15 patients, 8 of whom died; of the 7 patients who survived, 3 were neurologically intact, and 4 had suffered neurological damage;
- No infection occurred in 4 patients: 1 died due to ventricular bleeding, 1 survived intact, 1 survived with damage, 1 died from postoperative complications.

In this series, 52 patients were found whose injury was due to a pencil ($n = 41$), slate pencil ($n = 6$) or ballpoint pen ($n = 5$). In this group of 52 patients, several instances of penetration through the mouth, nose or temporal area were included. These will not be considered here, leaving a total of 40 TIPI cases:

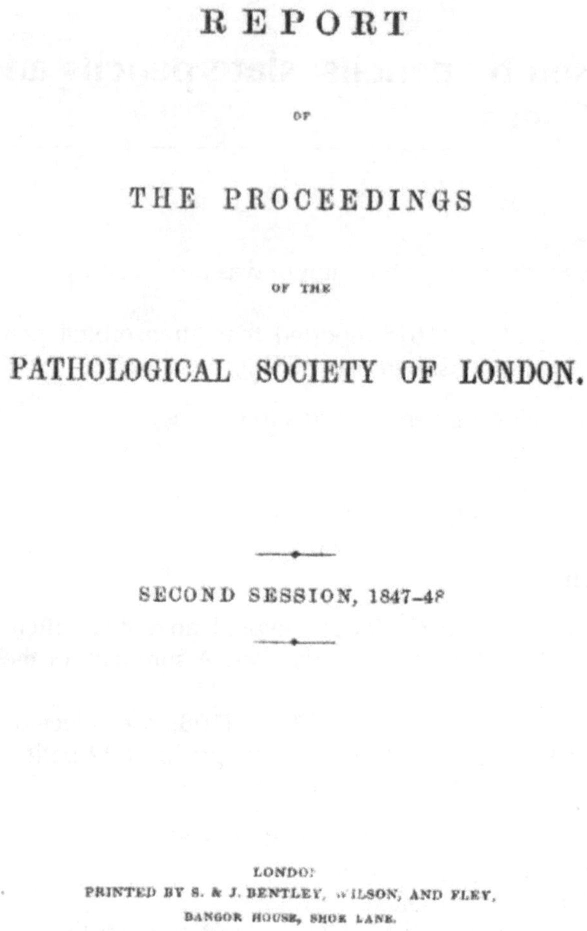

REPORT

OF

THE PROCEEDINGS

OF THE

PATHOLOGICAL SOCIETY OF LONDON.

SECOND SESSION, 1847–48

LONDON:
PRINTED BY S. & J. BENTLEY, WILSON, AND FLEY,
BANGOR HOUSE, SHOE LANE.

Figure 45 The earliest description of a TIPI caused by a pencil was produced by Hewitt in 1848 [312]

- 81% were under 10 years old (Miller *et al.* [108]: 74%; Bursick and Selker [202]: 82%; Kaiser *et al.* [238]: 85%);
- 64% were male (Miller: 68%; Bursick: 66%; Kaiser: 75%);
- 45% showed penetration through the upper eyelid (Miller: 58%);
- 80% were due to a fall;
- 73% involved the right orbit (Miller: 74%);
- 55% showed perforation of the orbital roof (Miller: 63%; Bursick: 72%);
- 55% infections occurred (practically always a brain abscess) (Miller: 79%);

- 40% overall mortality (Miller: 50%; Bursick: 36%);
- 100% mortality before 1944;
- 14% mortality after 1944 (antibiotics introduced) (Bursick: 22%);
- 40% infection rate after 1944 (in spite of antibiotics);
- 55% of survivors suffered permanent damage (Bursick: 50%), usually of the orbital structures, 17% showed persistent neurological damage (hemiplegia, behavioral disorders, epilepsy).

Since 1981, the infection rate has dropped drastically due to the introduction of CT/MRI facilities and immediate surgical intervention, preventing unnecessary further neurological deterioration.

Nevertheless, "the ordinary lead pencil is (still) a potentially lethal object" [202].

20

Suicide by TIPI

Self-inflicted eye injury does occur in psychiatric patients, the most serious one being auto-enucleation. Seven cases of attempted suicide involving a transorbital intracranially penetrating object could be traced. One more case has been added; here, the attempt involved penetration through the right nostril [79]. The references are:

1965 Murphree and Broussard [67]
1965 Albert *et al.* [161] (Figure 46)
1971 Bowen [309]
1977 Miller *et al.* [108]
1985 Yamamoto *et al.* [79]
1993 Greene *et al.* [264] (Figure 47)
1997 Lasky et al., case 1 [103] (Figure 48)
1997 Lasky *et al.*, case 2 [103]

The objects involved were:

Three ballpoint pens [67, 264, 309];
Three pencils [103 case 1, 108, 161];
One chopstick [79];
One toothbrush [103 case 2] (Figure 10).

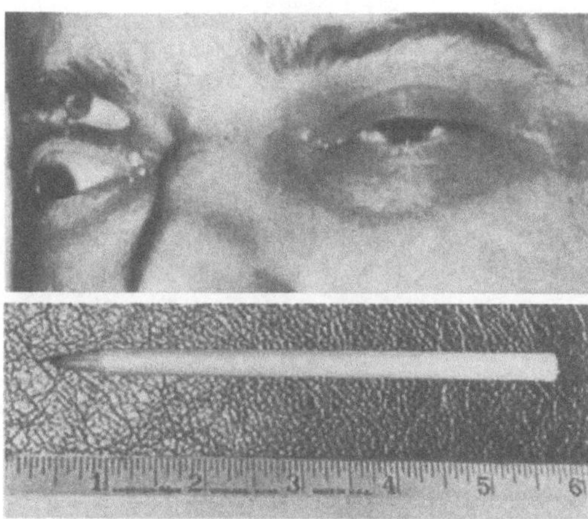

Figure 46 Pencil protruding from the orbit and pencil following removal

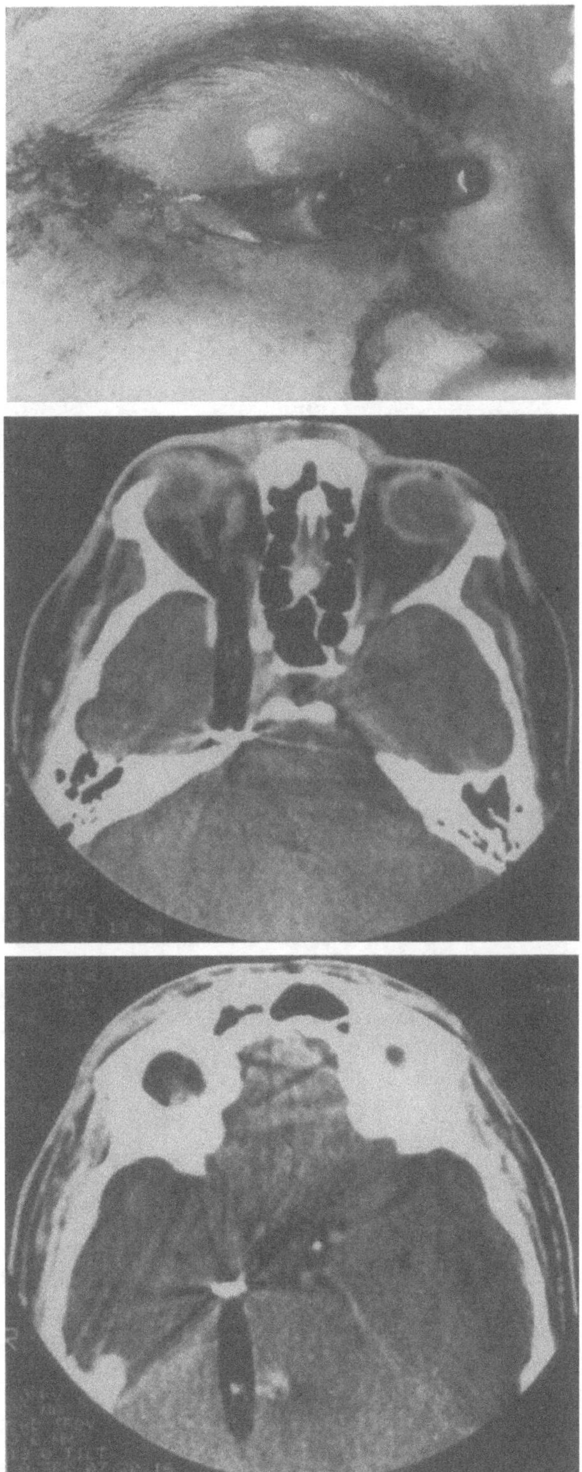

Figure 47 Protruding ballpoint pen penetrating into the posterior fossa, adjacent to the fourth ventricle. Local hemorrhage at the distal end of the pen

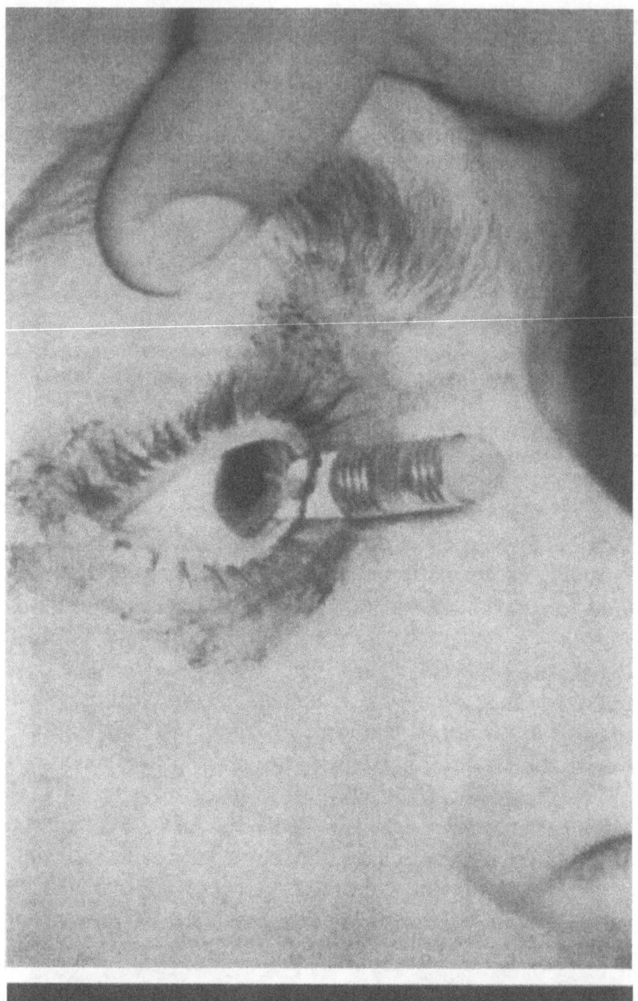

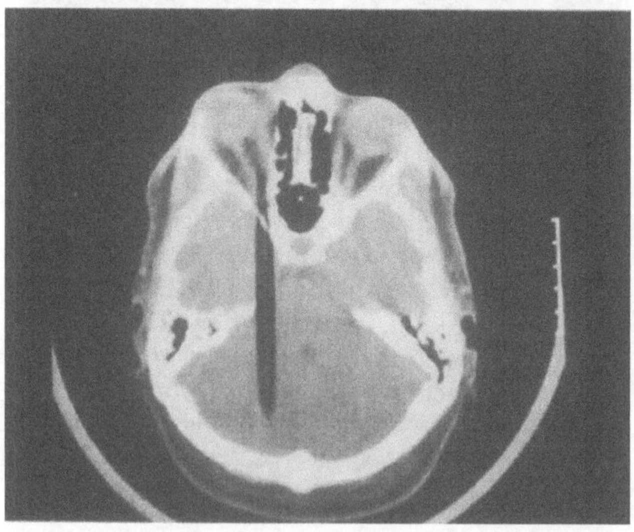

Figure 48 Protruding pencil, penetrating through the superior orbital fissure, terminating in the posterior fossa

Thus, there seems to be a preference for a ballpoint pen or pencil ($n=6$) as the agent in suicide attempts through the eye socket.

All 8 patients suffered from psychiatric disorders, such as depression and psychoses, and all were male.

Penetration always occurred through the right eye socket, with the exception of the case described by Yamamoto *et al.* [79], involving penetration through the right nostril. For right-handed persons, the right eye socket is a more convenient target. (It is assumed that all patients in this group were right-handed.)

Attempts to penetrate the left eye socket with an object held in the right hand are probably unsuccessful because this would lead to the head being turned to the left in an 'avoidance head turn' [103 case 2]. The sturdy lateral left orbital wall would then intercept the penetrating object and prevent intracranial penetration [103]. Nevertheless, the object can be deflected by this sturdy wall, finally reaching the intracranial space via the SOF.

The patient described by Greene *et al.* [264] had a "severe" contusion of the palmar surface of the right hand. Greene *et al.* attributed this bruising to "efforts to repeatedly drive the pen intracranially" (via the eye socket?). However, driving a pen through the medial SOF is easy and would not cause such a palm injury. The bruising could indicate that the penetrating ballpoint pen first hit the ala major before finally reaching the wider medial portion of the SOF. On the other hand, the bruising could have been caused by another preceding injury.

The ages of this group of 8 patients varied from 21 to 53 years. Penetration was usually attempted via the medial canthus ($n=4$) or the middle part of the upper eyelid ($n=1$). The eyeball remained intact in all cases, but, in 6 patients, there was an immediate loss of vision, usually combined with ophthalmoplegia. Intracranial penetration through the eye socket usually occurred via the SOF ($n=6$) but once via the ethmoid [309] and once via the sella [84].

Usually, the penetrating object was found still protruding from the eye socket ($n=6$) (Figures 46, 47 and 48).

The hollow shaft of a pen can allow the penetration of air intracranially, producing a pneumocephalus [67].

In one patient, the ballpoint pen lay so deep that it was only discovered on an X-ray. The patient had pushed the pen very deep into the right eye socket. In his report, Bowen [309] commented correctly that such a deep location ruled out a fall as a possible etiology; moreover, the patient showed contralateral conjunctival lacerations, indicating apparent unsuccessful attempts to push the pen in the left orbit.

In a TIPI due to a fall, part of the foreign body would still protrude from the eye socket and remain visible (see Chapter 17 on Fall injuries).

Naturally, what is possible in suicide can also occur in altercations or (attempted) murder. It is conceivable that a pencil, pushed deeply into an eye socket during a fight, is no longer visible but, as a rule, it remains palpable. Gates and Hardjasudarma [140] and Gottlieb *et al.* [144] (via the FOI) described such cases.

In attempted murder, however, the aggressor should be quite capable of pushing the pen deeper into the orbit, in an effort to cover up the penetrating object, thus masking aggression.

Despite suffering very deep self-inflicted penetration injuries, 6 patients were normally alert and co-operative. In 5 of these, no neurological disorders could be found. Two patients showed changes in consciousness and hemiplegia. Cranial nerve function disturbances were found in one patient. Temporary headache and vomiting were recorded. In one case, an asymptomatic traumatic dissection of the intracavernous carotid artery was revealed by angiography [264].

The surgical 'open and see' method was used twice; this involved complete trepanation to remove the foreign body retrogradely. The 'pull and see' method was applied six times, three times with CT monitoring, once with stand-by neurosurgical assistance and twice without. There were no complications, and only once did a CSF fistula arise [309]. One patient died due to meningitis 24 days after a deep brainstem injury [79]. The other patients survived their suicide attempt with the following defects:

- Blindness: 2 patients [67, 103 case 1];
- Blindness with ophthalmoplegia: 4 patients [103 case 2, 108, 161];
- Hemiparesis and optical nerve atrophy: 1 patient [309].

Stern [314] briefly reported the case of a patient who drove a pencil into the inner canthus. The resulting neurological disorder was a palatal myoclonus.

A self-inflicted transorbital injury can produce perforation of the ethmoidal sinus [313].

As a curiosity, the case described by Teeuw [315] is added.

A patient attempted suicide by sticking a ballpoint pen in each ear; the pens still protruded 3 cm. CT examination revealed that the pens had reached the parapharyngeal space in front of the spine, in-between the cartilage and bony part of the auditory meatus and under the mucous membrane, without causing any damage.

21
Mortality and morbidity

In the early literature, mortality rates were naturally very high, almost 100%.

For example, Winkfield [37] reported in 1877 that 17 of 18 patients with TIPI died.

In 1880, in the handbook by Graefe-Sämisch, Berlin reported a mortality of 80% (83% due to brain abscess and 11% to meningitis). Of the 20% survivors, one half suffered severe neurological damage [43]. However, these numbers also included patients with a penetrating injury near to the orbit.

In 1897, *The Lancet* [36] reported that, in the period 1886–1897, a mortality in excess of 90% was still associated with this injury.

Coqueret [20] noted in 1905 a mortality of at least 82%, three quarters due to meningitis or brain abscess.

In 1930, Birch-Hirschfeld [110] gave 12% as the mortality for all (including non-traversing) stab wounds involving the orbits.

After the turn of the century, a slight improvement in the prognosis occurred, as treatment changed from passive waiting to a more aggressive approach including trepanation with decompression and drainage [37, 44, 46].

After the Second World War, the prognosis improved significantly due to the introduction of antibiotics.

The percentages found by Miller *et al.* [108] in 1977 are well known, although they concern only wooden foreign bodies. His overall mortality was 45%; in the period before antibiotics, this percentage was 85%; in the antibiotic era, it dropped to 25%. Even with antibiotics, though, 64% of patients became infected.

In this series of patients, of those seen after 1977, 22% presented with an infection.

In Miller *et al.*'s series [108], 71% of 28 patients in the antibiotic era had surgery, with only two deaths. Of those who did not have an operation, only 38% survived (but this group undoubtedly included patients who were in poor condition and thus contraindicated for surgery).

Bard and Jarrett [12] noted a mortality of 25% in 1964. In 1981, Bursick and Selker [202] reported an overall mortality in their series of 36%. The mortality in their series before the introduction of antibiotics was 100%; after 1944, this dropped to 22%. Despite antibiotic treatment, 77% of patients developed infections after TIPI involving a pencil. Half of the survivors were left with permanent damage (loss of vision, optical nerve lesions, hemiparesis, epileptic seizures and behavioral disorders).

In 1980, Dietz [43] stated that the ratio of 80% mortality and 20% survival had now been reversed. Nowadays, 80% of patients are able to return to work [43].

Early recognition and treatment can increase the survival rate to 90% [108]. Thus, TIPI does not always have a negative outcome. If the orbital roof is perforated, injury to the frontal lobe can remain unnoticed, provided hemorrhage, infection or CSF loss does not occur [18]. If there is no serious damage to the brainstem and no acute massive hemorrhage, the injury can be treated, and the prognosis is potentially good [294].

In this series, the overall mortality was 26%. The mortality after perforation through the SOF was 15%, while that after perforation of the orbital roof with injury to the frontal lobe was twice as high (33%). Perforation via the medial canthus was associated with a higher mortality (24%) than perforation via the lateral canthus (15%). This supports Hoffman *et al.*'s hypothesis [47]: "Stab wounds of the orbit in the medial aspect of either the upper or lower eyelid are particularly dangerous."

Given modern developments, such as improved operating techniques, antibiotic therapy, CT and MRI, it is meaningful to evaluate the mortality rate over the past 20 years (1977–1997). We found a mortality of 13%.

Some 66% of patients underwent surgery. In 10%, the 'pull and see' method was used; only one patient died with an irreparable brainstem injury. The neurological condition of half of the remaining 'wait and see' group (24%) was too poor to undergo surgery.

Of all the surgically treated patients, only two died, one due to a generally poor condition. The other patient who died did not undergo surgery because

Table 4 A summary of the morbidity and mortality of 129 cases of TIPI in the period 1977–1997

13% mortality; 87% survivors

Treatment

Surgery:	66%; 2 deaths
Pull and see:	10%; 1 death
Wait and see:	24%; 13 deaths (poor condition)

16 patients died; 50% caused by umbrella TIPI

Condition of the survivors:

- 83% neurological recovery, but 28% remained with disturbances of vision and/or ocular nerves
- 12% severe neurological injury
- 2% moderate neurological disturbances
- 3% unknown

of untreatable lesions (destruction of the hypothalamus, ventricular hemorrhage, acute large hematoma, brainstem lesion, etc.).

Of the 16 patients who died, none evidenced obvious penetration through the SOF. In contrast, the orbital roof was clearly perforated in 6 cases, in 2 through the posterior part of the roof. In half of all fatal cases, the penetrating agent was an umbrella.

A further decrease in mortality is not to be expected, as the current level reflects serious irreparable damage.

Neurological restoration was achieved in 83% of the surviving patients, but 28% had vision and/or ocular nerve disturbances. Of those who survived, 12% suffered serious neurological damage; there was only slight damage in 2%, while the result was inconclusive in 3%.

22
Medicolegal aspects: prevention of TIPI

TIPI can have treacherous medicolegal implications for the treating physician [11].

As early as 1877, Annandale [41] pointed out that transorbital injuries with penetration through the conjunctiva could be invisible or hardly visible on the outside [316] even in the presence of extensive intracranial damage. In addition, he stressed that it is even easier to miss an intracranial injury when the object penetrates through the nose. The point of entry is hidden, or no connection is made between the slight injury and the serious clinical condition.

Clinically, this can sometimes lead to a completely wrong diagnosis, and, thus, (without autopsy) an incorrect cause of death is recorded. For example, a slight eye wound may not be associated with an intracerebral hematoma and the clinical diagnosis made is 'spontaneous intracerebral hematoma' although it was actually caused by a TIPI [311 case 2]. Only at autopsy (if done) is the TIPI discovered by finding a typical stab wound, suggesting a murder case [311]. Without autopsy, the true cause of death may be missed and a crime remain unsolved [7 case 1, 311 case 1].

In all cases of TIPI, the possibility that the injury was deliberately caused must be considered [190], as many are the result of aggression (Berlin 49%, Coqueret 44%, and this series 24%). Aggression should be suspected in the case of a comatose patient with a slight eye wound.

The (forensic) pathologist must always be aware that the cause of death can, unexpectedly, be a foreign body [282]. This may involve accidental injury in self-defence, in which the victim of an attack injures the attacker. For example, an umbrella may be used as a defensive weapon [20].

Occasionally, the remains of a foreign body are found in the wall of a brain abscess during an autopsy or operation, indicating an earlier, completely forgotten eye injury due to a fall, aggression or accident [7 case 8, 171, 176, 191, 261, 269, 282, 317]. Curiously enough, it is almost always the tip of a pencil which is found in these cases.

A correct diagnosis is of course of great therapeutic significance, as well as for insurance coverage later on [311].

Despite careful treatment by the physician, litigation will sometimes be unavoidable. Cases for litigation can involve the following:

1. A missed diagnosis; no link is made between the slight eye injury and the severe intracranial pathology [311], or the foreign body was not found [310]. The patient dies with 'only a slight eye wound'.

2. No adequate radiological examination was performed [11].
3. Surgical intervention did not lead to complete removal of the foreign body, and a (recurrent) brain abscess developed.
4. The patient is heavily intoxicated (drugs, alcohol) upon presentation and cannot be examined adequately. The physician decides to keep the patient under observation and wait for detoxification. Later, a neat pleasant ex-patient stands before the judge to press charges against the doctor: "The doctor was so busy that he (the patient) was not adequately examined soon after arrival nor medical records properly filled in" [11].
5. The development of (unavoidable) complications (blindness, personality changes, death, etc.).

Communication with the worried family is often limited due to the urgency of the situation and the admission of the patient to the Intensive Care Ward.

Therefore, make sure that extensive discussion is held regularly with the family; this can prevent much unpleasantness later. Record all details carefully in the medical record [11].

Once the initial examination has been completed, it is better to inform the patient and the family that remains of a foreign body may still be *in situ*, with the associated risks of inflammation, fistula formation and spontaneous extrusion [230]. This applies particularly to penetrating objects made of wood [239]. Such foreign bodies are difficult to locate and can remain undetected despite careful CT and MRI examination [239] (Chapter 11).

Complications due to remaining or undiscovered orbitocranial foreign bodies can suggest to the patient and his or her family (and the lawyer) that the treatment received was not up to current standards [239]. In all cases, the family and the patient must be informed that wood can be missed, and this warning should be recorded in the patient's files.

PREVENTION OF TIPI

In everyday life, there are many thin strong long objects which, in principle, could cause a TIPI. Certain toys for children should be labeled with a warning about the possibility of a fall TIPI, but this is not possible for every pen, pencil or slate pencil, although the packaging could be labeled. Children in kindergartens should be taught not to walk around while carrying such objects. Parents must raise their children in the same way [90].

23

Brief review of a patient series from the literature

A brief summary of each of the following references is given below.

Morrant Baker [7] 1888
Wertheim [19] 1904
Coqueret [20] 1905
Greig [9] 1924
Birch-Hirschfeld [110] 1930
McClure and Gardner [16] 1949
Kjer [10] 1954
Copper [24] 1957
Bullock *et al.* [18] 1959
Guthkelch [78] 1960
Unger and Umbach [59] 1963
Bard and Jarrett [12] 1964
Duffy and Bandari [116] 1969
De Villiers and Sevel [1] 1975
Dujovny *et al.* [258] 1975
Miller *et al.* [108] 1977
Yamaguchi *et al.* [153] 1978
Dietz [43] 1980
Bursick and Selker [202] 1981
Solomon *et al.* [71] 1993

Morrant Baker reviewed 12 cases from the literature and added one patient of his own: 12 men and 1 woman, all young except for one patient aged 73 years. Nine of them died; 2 of the 4 survivors did not suffer intracranial penetration. One patient survived with hemiplegia. In 7 cases, a brain abscess was the cause of death; in one, severe contusion and in one a carotid–cavernosus fistula (Nelaton's case; see Chapter 14 on Complications).

In his thesis, Wertheim published a detailed description of a personal case and a review of 11 cases from the literature. Of these latter, 5 could be traced [38–42] and were thus included in the current series, along with a case reported by Demours.

Wertheim included the case histories of:

1. Günther: a piece of wood penetrated through the inside of a child's upper eyelid. The child immediately developed convulsions and died after removal of the foreign body as a result of a hemorrhage. Autopsy revealed a penetrating injury through the SOF.
2. Faber: a 12-year-old boy was injured by a 7.5-cm-long piece of wood through the middle of the lower eyelid. He recovered without damage.
3. Hulke: a patient with an injury through the orbital roof died 3 weeks later due to a brain abscess.
4. Lawson and Johnson described penetrations, with objects 8.5 and 7 cm long, without symptoms.

Coqueret's work is considered in the chapter on historical aspects.

Greig reported one personal case and 23 cases from the literature. There were 18 men and 4 women. Most of the patients were under 28 years old; one patient was 46, while the ages of two were not recorded. Eight patients survived: 3 with good recovery, 5 with hemiplegia and mental disorders. In 13 cases, the injury occurred via the orbital roof and in 8, via the SOF. There were 4 brain abscesses – all of these patients died. Fifteen suffered a brain contusion, two hemorrhages, two meningitis and one suspected sepsis. Half of those with a brain contusion survived, probably because there was no infection, but practically all suffered serious neurological impairment.

Birch-Hirschfeld described 172 stab wounds of the orbit, both traversing and non-traversing, with 125 optical nerve injuries. Twenty patients died (3 from tetanus, 6 from carotid artery injury, 11 from meningitis). Curiously, no brain abscesses were recorded in his series. The mortality was 12% (but this low rate is due to the inclusion of non-traversing injuries). He cites 12 mostly transorbital injuries from the international literature, but, unfortunately, no references were provided, and are thus untraceable, with the exception of Ref. 25, Prokop cited in Ref. 84, and Ref. 109.

McClure and Gardner described 4 cases of their own, all male, ages ranging from 4 to 37 years. One involved a fall onto a pitchfork, leading only to transitory CSF leakage from the wound. In the second patient, a transitory SOF syndrome developed. The third patient suffered blindness and hemiplegia, while the fourth died of carotid artery hemorrhage with a CCF.

Kjer reported 15 patients, some with only an orbital injury. Only 4 transorbital injuries were described in detail. Nine patients suffered intracranial complications, 3 of whom first evidenced cerebral symptoms some time after admission, and thus after a symptom-free interval, with possibly initial transitory neurological symptoms, such as changes of consciousness, aphasia, etc. Three patients died. Seven patients were younger than 15 years old. None had an injured eyeball, and only 2 suffered visual symptoms. More than half had no radiological abnormalities, although a fracture was frequently found at operation. One patient died from tetanus. In 5 cases a craniotomy was performed. Twelve patients survived and returned to their usual activities; 4 of them were left with symptoms such as slight aphasia, paresis and epilepsy.

Copper described 4 patients, 2 boys and 2 girls, aged 3–12 years. They had all suffered from an injury received through the orbital roof, and thus associated with frontal lobe lesions. All underwent surgery, 3 acutely and one after recurrent meningitis. They all recovered; in 2 of them a Torkildson operation was necessary.

Bullock *et al.* published accounts of 5 cases, all children younger than 10 years, 4 boys and 1 girl. One died, and 2 of the 4 survivors suffered serious disability.

Guthkelch described 6 patients aged 2–9 years, 5 injured by a fall trauma. All of them suffered a perforation of the orbital roof, with no initial changes of consciousness. Four developed late infections (3 with brain abscess, 1 with meningitis).

One patient died, 4 recovered. One suffered a bilateral frontal lobe lesion due to a large hematoma and was left with epilepsy and personality changes. Three patients required several operations and a long hospital stay.

Unger and Umbach reported 5 cases. Four were aged 6–9 years and the fifth was 65 years old; this patient died later on due to other causes. Three of these cases were fall injuries. In 2 cases the injury did not reach the intracranial contents. Two injuries penetrated through the orbital roof and 2 probably through the SOF. The surviving 4 patients recovered, one with a bilateral visual deficit.

Bard and Jarrett described 9 personal patients. In 8 cases, a radiological examination was carried out but only one patient showed a fracture. Two patients died of intracerebral hemorrhage and contusion; the seriousness of the injury had not been recognized. Five developed fulminant or insidious meningitis and an abscess totally unexpectedly after an orbital injury. Two developed a CSF fistula and pneumocephalus, revealing the existence of intracranial penetration. Four suffered loss of vision.

In addition, Bard reviewed 44 cases from the literature: 11 died, and of the 33 survivors, 11 were blind in one eye. Of these 44 cases, in 16 cases the diagnosis first became evident after 24 h, with the appearance of cerebral symptoms; in 12 of these 16, this symptom-free period lasted a week or more. In 19 of the 44 patients, radiological examination revealed some evidence of penetration. In 15 cases the results were negative, but, in 5 of these, the clinical course suggested intracranial penetration. In 10 patients, radiological exam revealed no abnormalities.

Duffy and Bandari presented 6 cases (one high-velocity and 2 air gun pellet injuries are not included here). In 3 cases, a fall TIPI was involved. In 5 cases, the injury penetrated the orbital roof and in one probably via the SOF.

There were 2 immediate complications: one ventricular hemorrhage and one hemorrhage of the anterior cerebral artery; both patients died. The 4 late complications were a CCF, 2 brain abscesses and one recurrent meningitis.

Three patients survived without symptoms, while one suffered severe neurological impairment.

De Villiers and Sevel described 10 cases, all more than 20 years old, and all were TIPI cases resulting from direct aggression.

Six patients suffered an eye injury, 4 of which were serious; 3 of the latter did not survive the attack.

In 3 cases, meningitis developed, and, in 5, the carotid artery was injured (2 CCF, 2 traumatic aneurysms, one carotid artery occlusion).

In 7 cases, the foreign body was a knife, in one case a pencil. In all, 3 died. No late infections were noted.

Dujovny *et al.* published 2 personal cases, showing a good recovery after surgery. They also reviewed 50 cases from the literature of which 9 patients died and 13 survived the trauma with a permanent unilateral loss of vision. Twenty-nine were younger than 12 years old.

Early appearing complications included: hemorrhage, contusions, and large vessel lesions. In 7 cases, meningitis and/or brain abscesses developed.

The late morbidity showed: CCF ($n = 4$), CSF fistula ($n = 7$), epilepsy ($n = 4$), ophthalmoplegia ($n = 9$), hemiplegia ($n = 4$) and pneumocephalus ($n = 5$).

Radiological examination revealed abnormalities in 19 cases, while, in 18 cases, no indications of a fracture were found.

Miller *et al.* reported one case of an attempted suicide with a pencil, as well as a significant review of 42 cases of TIPI involving sharp wooden objects, collected from the literature and published in the period 1834–1975.

In all, 80% of the patients were younger than 20 years old; indeed the majority were younger than 10 years old. The ratio men to women was 3 : 1. There was not a single eyeball injury, and usually the right eye-socket was involved. Intracranial injury was suspected immediately in only 26%, based on acute intracranial symptoms.

Neurological disorders developed rapidly in 29%, while, after 1 week, this proportion had risen to 60%. In the remaining 40%, the interval lasted between 2 weeks and 13 years (2/5 longer than 1 year).

A pencil was involved most often ($n = 19$), causing 15 cases of inflammation, 12 involving a brain abscess.

Radiological examination was performed on 25 patients: 72% of the results indicated an abnormality. Often, the radiographs were taken only after cerebral symptoms had developed.

Penetration occurred through the orbital roof in 71%, 10% via the SOF and 5% via the lamina cribrosa. There was not a single injury running through the optical foramen, although often an optical nerve lesion occurred.

Pieces of wood were not suspected but were present in 92% of 37 patients, and were eventually demonstrated. Occasionally, the wood was only revealed in the abscess wall microscopically.

The morbidity was 75% and included nerve impairment, motor and sensibility disorders, epileptic seizures, hydrocephalus and mental disorders.

The overall mortality was 45%. Miller *et al.* correctly distinguished between mortality before the introduction of antibiotics (85%) and afterwards (25%).

In the pre-antibiotic era, 78% of patients developed an infection (of whom 58% brain abscess, 25% meningitis); there were also 8% vascular abnormalities and 8% unknown. In the antibiotic era, 64% still developed an infection (of whom 57% brain abscess, 14% meningitis) and 29% developed hemorrhage. In total, infections developed in 69% of the cases, with brain abscess in 48%, usually caused by staphylococci.

Of the 28 patients in the antibiotic era, 71% underwent surgery, and of these only 2 died. In the antibiotic era, 90% of patients survived after surgery and 38% without surgery. However, this latter group most likely includes seriously injured patients who were not expected to survive or were inoperable.

Early surgery was associated with 33% morbidity; late surgery with 50%.

Yamaguchi *et al.* summarized 73 patients from the literature and 2 personal cases. From the English summary, the following is cited.

Mostly males and usually children were injured. Orbital intracranial injury had a higher mortality than intracranial penetration via another route. The causes of death were: brain contusion, intracerebral hemorrhage, subdural hematoma and meningitis.

In 63% a frontal lobe lesion was found (according to [65]).

Dietz reviewed 12 cases (3 high-velocity injuries are not considered here).

Eight patients with TIPI developed acute symptoms: 5 CSF fistula, 6 brain lesions. There were no cases of acute infection. In 4 cases, late complications arose, after a few months to 14 years: in 4 cases, recurrent meningitis; in 3, a brain abscess occurred.

Bursick and Selker produced a significant review of more than 22 cases of TIPI caused by pencils, 'the pencil puncture injury'.

In 82%, the patient was under 10 years of age; none was older than 24 years. More than two thirds of the patients were male.

In 4 cases, symptoms appeared immediately, and, in the remainder, after days or years; 33% first developed symptoms 1 year or more after the trauma. In 72%, penetration occurred through the orbital roof, less frequently via the lamina cribrosa or temporal region.

Overall mortality was 36%. Before 1944, i.e. before the sulphonamide–antibiotics era, the mortality was 100% (4 deaths due to meningitis or a brain abscess). After 1944, the mortality dropped to 22%: 4 deaths (3 due to brain abscesses, 1 to vascular injury). Despite the administration of antibiotics, infection developed in 77% of patients.

Half of the survivors suffered permanent disability, vision loss, optical atrophy, ophthalmoplegia, hemiparesis, epileptic seizures and behavioral disorders. In general, these disabilities did not develop as a direct result of the trauma, but rather due to subsequent infection and thus may have been partly preventable.

Solomon *et al.* described 5 cases: 3 male, 1 female and a child (sex not stated); 2 were 18, one was 22 and 2 were 1 year old.

In 4 cases, the injury penetrated through the orbital roof, once through both the orbital floor and roof. Conservative treatment and, in one case, a shunt operation led to good results in 4 patients. One patient underwent intracranial surgery.

List of patients

Year	Author	Gender	Age	Reference	Object	Aggression	Fall injury	Accident	Suicide attempt	Orbit (R/L)
1818	Demours	?	10	Cited in 19 and 20, obs. 193	Point of spinning machine			+		?
1824	Cooper	f	12	Cited in 9	Scissors		+			?
1832	Anonymous	m	15	318	Pipe stem	+				L
1834	Scott	m	16	33	Foil			+		R
1834	Scott	m	10	33	Broom			+		L
1837	MacFarlane	m	57	20, obs. 187	Piece of iron	+				L
1838	Selwyn	m	4	319	Knife		+			R
1847	Decaisne	m	?	20, obs. 193	Ramrod			+		R
1847	Gintrac	?	12	20, obs. 153	Knife		+			L
1848	Hewitt	f	2	312	Pencil		+			R
1851	Little	m	28	100	Red hot iron rod	+				L
1852	Montgomery	m	15	20, obs. 228	Pitchfork			+		L
1853	Guthrie	m	9	Cited in 9	Wire			+		R
1853	Guthrie	f	?	Cited in 9	Pipe stem	+				L
1854	Mackenzie W	m	?	Cited in 9	Umbrella	+				L
1855	Jamieson	m	?	101	Walking stick ferrule	+?				R
1855	Nélaton	m	21	Cited in 7, 199	Umbrella	+				L
1859	Fritz	Child	2	Cited in 20, obs. 234	Pipe stem			+		L
1864	Pagenstecher	f	7	42	Knitting needle		+			R
1867	Lawson	m	?	Cited in 9	Umbrella	+				L
1869	Betke	f	1¼	35	Spout of oilcan		+			R
1872	La Force	m	10	38	Piece of wood		+?			?

1877	Annandale	f	14	41	Knitting needle			+		L
1879	Bower	m	45	320	Umbrella	+				L
1879	Steavenson	m	21	67	Knitting needle			+		L
1882	Donkin	m	12	321	Steel rib of umbrella			+		R
1882	Prideaux	m	12	117	Wooden stick			+		R
1884	Jackson	m	7	316	Piece of wood		+			L
1885	Gaboriau	f	19	Cited in 20, obs. 108	Umbrella	+				L
1886	Hawkins	?	3	Cited in 36	Knitting needle		+			R
1886	Pope	m	37	20, obs. 18	Umbrella	+				L
1888	Morrant Baker	m	26	7	Stick	+				L
1888	Morrant Baker	m	?	7	Stick	+				L
1888	Morrant Baker	m	?	7	Umbrella	+				L
1888	Morrant Baker	m	?	7	?	+2				R
1888	Morrant Baker	m	3	7	?		+			R
1888	Morrant Baker	f	6	7	Slate pencil		+			R
1888	Morrant Baker	m	?	7	Pen holder and nib	?	?	?	?	R
1889	Bouton fils	m	?	Cited in 20, obs. 175	Umbrella	+				L
1890	Lotz	f	3½	40	Slate pencil		+			R, via cheek
1891	Laplace	m	10	45	Fencing foil		+			L
1891	Polaillon	m	18	44	Umbrella		+			L
1894	Johnson	m	49	322	Splinter of wood			+		R
1895	De Nobele	m	?	62	Umbrella	+				L
1895	De Nobele	m	?	62	Pipe stem	+				L
1896	Adamük	m	?	39	Branch			+		R
1897	Bramwell	m	9	70	Iron rod		+			R
1897	Winkfield	m	12	37	Ferrule end of fishing rod		+			R

Year	Author	Gender	Age	Reference	Object	Aggression	Fall injury	Accident	Suicide attempt	Orbit (R/L)
1898	Koster	?	?	323	Pipe stem	?	?	?		?
1898	McEwan	f	8	20, obs. 90	Cane	?	?	?		R
1899	Rockliffe and Hainworth	m	28	324	Pipe stem	+				L
1900	Arloing	m	28	20, obs 163	Pitchfork			+		L
1900	Martial	m	46	63	Fencing foil			+		R
1900	Mackenzie	m	?	20, obs. 128	Pitchfork			+		?
1900±	Rohmer	m	14	20, obs. 270	Pitchfork			+		L
1901	Nuel	m	14	199	Umbrella	+				L
1902	Socquet	m	41	20, obs. 12	Umbrella	+				L
1902	Socquet	m	?	20, obs. 14	Umbrella	+				R
1902	Socquet	m	?	20, obs. 309	Umbrella	+				L
1904	Mauclaire and Socquet	m	45	20, obs. 18	Umbrella	+				L
1904	Wertheim	m	42	19	Branch		+			L
1907	Casali	m	?	325	Umbrella		+?			L
1914	v.d. Hoeve	m	?	326	Knife	+				Both orbitae
1914	Solieri	f	17	64	Umbrella			+		R, via nose
1914	Solieri	m	4	64	Pitchfork			+		R
1923	Gatchell	m	?	85	Pipe stem	+				L
1924	Greig	m	12	9	Umbrella rib		+			L
1928	Walchshofer	f	16	96	Pitchfork			+		R
1929	Haase	?	4	84	Ruler		+			R
1929	Prokop	m	8	Cited in 84	Pitchfork			+		L
1932	Anonymous	m	?	327	Hook			+		R
1932	Key and McCrammen	m	3	307	Pen holder		+			Via mouth
1933	Canuyt *et al.*	f	11	328	Branch			+ playing		L
1934	Davis	m	12	176	Slate pencil		+			Nose
1935	Meyer and Roeting	m	10	329	Piece of wood		+			L
1937	Baron	m	10½	91	Brake handle		+			R
1938	Kuntzman	?	5	330	Slate pencil		+			R

1941	Frieman	m	32	331	Metal splinter			+	R
1941	Kumano	m	7	332	Aluminium rod			+	R
1942	Thomas	m	16	333	Knife	+			L, not intracranial
1944	Slaughter and Alvis	f	3	283	Pencil		+		R
1947	Rees	m	3	334	Branch		+		L
1948	Klotz	f	7	268	Pencil		+		?
1948	Palin	m	?	87	Piece of ice			+	?
1948	Swoboda	m	10	76	Theatre sword			+	R
1949	McClure and Gardner	m	4	16	Pitchfork		+		L
1949	McClure and Gardner	m	18	16	Grass stubble		+		L
1949	McClure and Gardner	m	37	16	Wooden splinter			+	R
1949	McClure and Gardner	m	22	16	Knife	+			L
1949	Rowbotham	Child	?	15	Stick		+		?
1949	Rowbotham	?	?	15	Piece of wood			+	?
1950	Flieringa	m	?	173	Pen holder	+			?
1951	Field	m	7	168	Curtain rod		+		L orbit→ pharynx
1952	Le Win	f	1½	86	Tea spoon		+		R
1952	Muscas	f	14	281	Knife		+		L
1952	Muscas	m	36	281	Piece of wood			+	R
1952	Schneider and Henderson	m	27	56	Ice pick	+			L
1953	Sedan and Pailas	m	21	115	Metal rod			+	R
1954	Carver *et al.*	m	19	253	Wooden stick			+	R
1954	Kjer	m	46	10	Peat fork			+	R

Year	Author	Gender	Age	Reference	Object	Aggression	Fall injury	Accident	Suicide attempt	Orbit (R/L)
1954	Kjer	m	3	10	Peg		+			R
1954	Kjer	m	16	10	Pitchfork		+			L
1954	Kjer	m	6	10	Pitchfork			+		L
1954	Platt	f	3	272	Pitchfork			+		R
1955	Cartwright *et al.*	f	9	203	Branch		+			R, not intracranial
1956	Larmande *et al.*	m	23	197	Fencing foil			+		R
1956	Medler	f	13	186	Piece of wood			+		R
1957	Copper	f	3½	24	Ground peg		+			R
1957	Copper	m	9	24	Stick		+ playing			R
1957	Copper	f	3	24	Stick		+ playing			L
1957	Copper	m	12	24	Branch			+ thrown		L
1958	de Grood and Goettsch	m	20	22	Knife	+?				L
1959	Bullock *et al.*	f	7½	18	Steel rod			+		L
1959	Bullock *et al.*	m	7	18	Stick			+ playing		R
1959	Bullock *et al.*	m	9	18	Sled runner			+		L
1959	Bullock *et al.*	m	10	18	Pitchfork			+		R
1959	Bullock *et al.*	m	9	18	Arrow		+			R
1959	Lavergne	m	65	17	Gear stick		+			R
1960	Guthkelch	f	9	78	Bamboo stick		+			L
1960	Guthkelch	m	9	78	Iron spike		+			R
1960	Guthkelch	m	6	78	?		+			R
1960	Guthkelch	f	2	78	Pencil		+			R
1960	Guthkelch	m	2	78	Chisel		+			R
1960	Guthkelch	f	7	78	Coat rack			+		R
1961	Goald and Ronderos	m	46	198	Steel spring			+		R, cheek
1961	Klug and Tzonas	m	27	266	Metal rod			+		L
1961	Lehmann	m	14	335	Pitchfork			+		R
1962	Kreft and Duffy	m	22	66	Piece of metal			+		R

1962	Unger and Umbach	f	9	59	Slate pencil		+			R
1962	Unger and Umbach	m	6	59	Slate pencil		+			L
1962	Unger and Umbach	m	7	59	Nail			+		R
1962	Unger and Umbach	m	9	59	Fence			+		L
1962	Unger and Umbach	m	65	59	Glass splinter		+			R
1963	Blumberg and Johnston	m	20	282	Pencil		+?			R
1964	Bard and Jarrett	m	28	12	Knife	+				R
1964	Bard and Jarrett	m	7	12	Sled runner			+		L
1964	Bard and Jarrett	m	43	12	Umbrella	+				R
1964	Bard and Jarrett	m	53	12	Steel wire			+		L
1964	Bard and Jarrett	m	36	12	Knife	+				L
1964	Bard and Jarrett	m	35	12	Knife	+				R
1964	Bard and Jarrett	m	3	12	Pencil		+?			R
1964	Bard and Jarrett	m	54	12	? Puncture wound			+ automobile		R
1964	Bard and Jarrett	m	29	12	Knife	+				L
1964	Bickerstaff	m	6	300	Stick		+			Via mouth
1964	Bickerstaff	m	4	300	Pencil		+			Via mouth
1964	Horner *et al.*	m	4	171	Pencil		+			R, temp
1964	Horner *et al.*	m	4½	171	Pencil		+			L, temp
1964	Horner *et al.*	m	20	171	Pencil		+?			R
1964	Markham *et al.*	m	11	304	Car antenna		+			Via mouth, intracranial
1964	Markham *et al.*	m	17	304	Car antenna		+			R
1964	Wuttke	m	3½	49	Iron rod		+			R
1965	Albert *et al.*	m	27	161	Pencil				+	R
1965	Henyer and Passmore	f	2	287	Pencil		+			L, not intracranial
1965	Lalla and Pillai	f	19	336	Umbrella		+			R
1965	Mansuy *et al.*	m	3	72	Glass rod		+			L
1965	Murphree and Broussard	m	21	67	Ballpoint pen				+	R
1966	Cressman and Hayes	m	34	247	Antenna jeep		+			L

Year	Author	Gender	Age	Reference	Object	Aggression	Fall injury	Accident	Suicide attempt	Orbit (R/L)
1966	Ho *et al.*	m	7	166	Pruned rose bush		+			L, sinus maxillaris
1966	De Grood	f	5	23	Pencil			+?		L
1967	Gossman	m	24	163	Umbrella ferrule	+				L
1967	Stöwsand	f	47	267	Knife	+				L
1969	Duffy and Bandari	f	2½	116	Pencil		+			L
1969	Duffy and Bandari	m	56	116	Wire			+		R
1969	Duffy and Bandari	m	2½	116	Pencil		+			R
1969	Duffy and Bandari	m	2	116	Screwdriver		+			R
1969	Duffy and Bandari	f	8½	116	Knitting needle			+		L
1969	Duffy and Bandari	m	27	116	Knife	+				R
1969	Walsh and Hoyt	m	18	293	Knife	+				L
1970	Boschetti and Bellandi	m	32	337	Nail			+		R
1970	Sarda *et al.*	?	2½	113	Branch		+			L, not intracranial
1971	Bowen	m	44	309	Pencil				+	R
1971	Gouazé and Santini	m	51	58	Metal rod			+		R
1971	Gouazé and Santini	m	40	58	Pitchfork			+		L
1971	Jackson *et al.*	m	23	149	Knife	+				L, via lateral orbital wall
1971	Lee and Lin	m	35	139	Knife	+				R
1971	Schmidt and Frowein	m	3	155	Twig			+		L
1971	Schmidt and Frowein	m	9	155	Iron rod		+			R
1971	Schmidt and Frowein	m	50	155	Knife	+				L
1971	Schmidt and Frowein	f	18	155	Pitchfork			+		L

1971	Wronski and Tota	f	7	317	Pencil		+?		R
1972	Di Maio and Di Maio	m	42	338	Knife	+			L
1972	Kessler	m	14	164	Pitchfork			+	L
1973	Klug	f	2½	88	Welding rod		+?		L
1973	Klug	m	35	88	Gear stick			+	L
1973	Klug	m	20	88	Ski stick			+	R
1973	Merritt *et al.*	m	32	109	Spring			+	L
1973	Noterman *et al.*	m	49	92	Plastic handle			+	L
1973	Siedschlag and Feldman	f	33	339	Glass fragments			+	R
1973	Stadler *et al.*	f	2	269	Pencil		+		R
1973	Thomson et al.	m	8	102	Tent-pole spike	?	?	?	L
1974	Decroix and Pendriel	m	21	200	TV antenna			+	L
1975	De Villiers and Sevel	m	?	1	Wire			+?	R
1975	De Villiers and Sevel	m	31	1	Knife	+			L
1975	De Villiers and Sevel	m	?	1	Stick	+			R
1975	De Villiers and Sevel	m	40	1	Knife	+			L
1975	De Villiers and Sevel	m	20	1	Knife	+			L
1975	De Villiers and Sevel	m	30	1	Knife	+			R
1975	De Villiers and Sevel	m	30	1	Knife	+			L
1975	De Villiers and Sevel	m	25	1	Knife	+			L
1975	De Villiers and Sevel	m	23	1	Knife	+			R
1975	De Villiers and Sevel	f	25	1	Pencil	+			L

Year	Author	Gender	Age	Reference	Object	Aggression	Fall injury	Accident	Suicide attempt	Orbit (R/L)
1975	De Villiers and Sevel	f	25	1	Pencil	+				L
1975	Dujovny *et al.*	m	10	258 + 13	Pencil		+			L
1975	Dujovny *et al.*	m	8	258 + 13	Iron rod		+			L
1975	Gralek and Mert	m	47	340	Twig			+		?
1975	Patten	m	66	210	Piece of wood			+		R
1975	Bullier *et al.*	m	38	278	Rib of umbrella			+		L
1976	Bullier *et al.*	f	34	278	Rib of umbrella		+			R
1976	Fanning *et al.*	f	4	254	Pencil		+			L
1976	Vérin *et al.*	f	Child	189	Wooden toy sword			+		R
1976	Vérin *et al.*	m	9	189	Arrow			+		L
1977	Kupusarevic	m	28	165	Branch			+		L, via orbital to sinus maxillaris
1977	Lunsford *et al.*	m	9	213	Stick		+			R
1977	Miller *et al.*	m	24	108	Pencil				+	R
1977	Mohssenipour and Twerdy	m	10	162	Knife		+			L
1977	Rahman *et al.*	m	30	174	Nail			+		R
1977	Rahman *et al.*	m	40	174	Metal piece			+		R
1978	Carothers	m	25	251	Umbrella	+				R
1978	Carothers	m	29	251	Umbrella	+				L
1978	Shima *et al.*	f	47	277	Bamboo stick		+			R
1978	Tomita and Miwa	f	2	112	Screwdriver		+			R, via os frontale
1978	Tomita and Miwa	m	2	112	Knitting needle	?	?	?		R
1978	Tomita and Miwa	m	3	112	Chopstick	?	?	?		L
1978	Von Dellen and Lipschitz	f	23	53	Knife	+				L
1978	Windle Taylor	m	15	105	Harpoon			+		R, ...

1978	Yamaguchi *et al.*	m	49	153	Piece of wood			+	L
1978	Yamaguchi *et al.*	m	18	153	?			+	L
1978	McCabe *et al.*	m	10	29	Needle-fish			+	R
1979	Gonçalves da Silva and Gonçalves da Silva	m	38	158	Knife	+			R
1979	Stewart and Polomeno	f	8	196	Branch		+		R
1979	de Tribolet *et al.*	m	8	175	Paint brush		+		R, via nose
1980	Aichmair	m	?	188	?	+			?
1980	Brock	m	40	245	Branch			+	L
1980	Foy and Sharr	m	1	270	Pencil		+		R
1980	Foy and Sharr	m	6	270	Pencil		+		R
1980	Foy and Sharr	m	3	270	Pencil		+		R, temporal
1980	Healy	m	22	188	Billiard cue	+			L, via nose
1980	Kazarian *et al.*	m	8	208	Piece of wood		+		R
1980	Yougshu and Guojun	m	32	141	Glass splinter			+	L
1980	Yougshu and Guojun	m	4	141	Chopstick		+		L
1981	Bursick and Selker	m	1	202	Pencil		+		R
1981	Girouard *et al.*	m	8	246	Tentpole			+	L
1981	Kitahara *et al.*	m	10	297	Umbrella	+			L
1981	Kitahara *et al.*	m	27	297	Umbrella	+			L
1981	Kitahara *et al.*	m	38	297	Umbrella	+			L
1981	Kitahara *et al.*	f	1	297	Chopstick		+		R
1981	Kitahara *et al.*	m	20	297	Piece of wood			+	R
1981	Kitahara *et al.*	f	54	297	Umbrella		+		R
1981	Nagahiro *et al.*	m	30	291	Chopstick	+			R
1982	Amano and Kamano	m	7	81	Bamboo		+		L
1982	Dabezies *et al.*	m	15	69	Afro comb	+			L, via lateral orbital wall

Year	Author	Gender	Age	Reference	Object	Aggression	Fall injury	Accident	Suicide attempt	Orbit (R/L)
1982	Healy	m	51	341	Knife	+				L
1982	Hungerford	m	22	185	Fencing foil			+		R
1983	Doucet *et al.*	m	19	193	Piece of wood			+		R
1983	Guttierrez *et al.*	m	29	104	Harpoon			+		L
1983	Hoffman *et al.*	m	41	47	Umbrella	+				L
1983	Kaiser *et al.*	m	1½	238	Pencil		+			R, temporal
1983	Siegel *et al.*	m	41	156	Umbrella	+				L
1983	Weisman *et al.*	m	4	151	Stick		+			R
1984	Anderson *et al.*	m	4	93	Spout of oilcan		+			L
1984	Krüger *et al.*	m	42	342	Steel pipe			+		R
1984	Nath *et al.*	f	31	265	Knife	+				R
1985	Bullock and van Dellen	m	24	194	Knife	+				L
1985	Chapman and Grove	m	9	6	Curtain rod, thrown			+		L
1985	Chapman and Grove	m	9	6	Umbrella		+			R
1985	Inbasekaran *et al.*	m	10	179	Pencil		+?			Via nose
1985	Yamamoto *et al.*	m	35	79	Chopstick				+	R, via nose
1986	Kirkby	m	?	343	Billiard cue		+			R
1986	Mono *et al.*	f	5½	75	Arrow			+		R
1986	Mono *et al.*	m	13	75	Wire rod		+			R
1986	MacEwen and Fullerton	f	28	189	Knife	+				R
1986	Nakayama *et al.*	m	17	65	Bamboo stick		+			R
1986	Quayle	m	59	184	Ballpoint pen		+			L, not intracranial
1986	Sebag *et al.*	m	5	187	TV antenna		+			R
1986	Sebag *et al.*	m	2½	187	Pencil		+			R
1986	Sebag *et al.*	m	17	187	Umbrella	+				R
1987	Braun *et al.*	m	6	234	Branch			+		L

1987	McHugh *et al.*	m	47	215	Branch		+		R
1987	Rahimizadeh *et al.*	f	5	82	Piece of glass	?	?	?	L
1987	Ravelli *et al.*	m	29	344	Steel hook			+	L
1988	Charteris	m	2	20	Ballpoint pen		+		R, not intracranial
1988	Hansen *et al.*	m	7	146	Twig			+	L
1988	Kadota *et al.*	f	38	345	Chopstick	+			R
1988	Vander and Nelson	m	20	83	Nail			+	L
1988	Yamashita *et al.*	f	38	80	Chopstick	+			R
1989	Sollmann *et al.*	m	42	119	Metal pipe			+	R
1989	Mains and Nagle	m	5½	31	Dowel		+		Via mouth
1990	Lawson *et al.*	m	19	89	Kangaroo tooth			+	R
1990	Scarfo *et al.*	m	29	50	Nail			+	R
1990	Scarfo *et al.*	m	43	50	Metal fragment			+	L, via sinus maxillaris
1990	Tokitsu *et al.*	m	24	177	Umbrella	+			L
1990	Tokitsu *et al.*	m	29	177	Umbrella	+			R, via nose
1991	Jones *et al.*	m	41	275	Plant stem			+	R
1991	Kane *et al.*	f	72	98	Motorbike stand		+		R
1991	Khalil *et al.*	m	12	294	Metal rod	+			R
1991	Khalil *et al.*	m	79	294	Knife?	+			L
1991	Mutlukan *et al.*	m	41	152	Wooden foliage		+		R
1991	Sarvesvaran	m	29	310	Umbrella	+			R
1991	Vlková and Slapák	m	35	68	Twig		+		R
1991	Vlková and Slapák	m	66	68	Door handle		+		R
1991	Zentner *et al.*	m	12	157	Wooden stick		+		R
1992	Fallon *et al.*	f	2½	178	Wooden stick		+		R, via nose
1992	Gottlieb *et al.*	m	27	144	Pencil	+			L
1992	Swanson and Augustine	m	47	128	Fish hook			+	L
1992	Shevach *et al.*	m	10	286	Umbrella		+		L
1992	Specht *et al.*	m	9	77	Golf tee		+		R

Year	Author	Gender	Age	Reference	Object	Aggression	Fall injury	Accident	Suicide attempt	Orbit (R/L)
1993	Agarwal *et al.*	m	8	114	Piece of wood			+ playing		L
1993	Agarwal *et al.*	m	9	114	Pencil		+			R
1993	Bank and Carolan	m	5	90	Piece of wood		+			R
1993	Coro *et al.*	f	3	148	Pencil		+			L
1993	Devi *et al.*	m	26	249	Saw blade			+		L
1993	Devi *et al.*	m	31	249	Iron rod			+		L
1993	Gates and Hardjasudarma	m	22	140	Pencil	+				R
1993	Greene *et al.*	m	34	264	Ballpoint pen				+	R
1993	Michon *et al.*	m	11	60, 74	Metal rod			+		R
1993	Oguz *et al.*	m	7	160	Pencil		+			R
1993	Rao *et al.*	m	44	143	Stick		+			L
1993	Solomon *et al.*	m	18	71	Billiard cue			+		R
1993	Solomon *et al.*	f	1½	71	Scissors		+			R
1993	Solomon *et al.*	m	22	71	Twig		+			L
1993	Solomon *et al.*	?	1	71	Screwdriver		+			R
1993	Solomon *et al.*	m	18	71	Pool cue			+?		L
1993	Shrivas and Kinzha	m	8	145	Stick			+		R
1994	Betz *et al.*	m	26	311	Umbrella	+				L
1994	Betz *et al.*	m	?	311	Umbrella		+			R
1994	Ersahin *et al.*	m	5	263	Nail		+			L
1994	Heyworth *et al.*	m	26	142	Billiard cue	+				L
1994	Ildan *et al.**	m	7	261	Pencil		+			R
1994	O'Neill *et al.*	m	25	55	Arrow			+		R
1994	Stern	m	28	314	Billiard cue	+				L
1994	Sato *et al.*	?	1	346	Ballpoint pen	?	?	?		L
1994	Sato *et al.*	?	1	346	Chopstick	?	?	?		R
1994	Sato *et al.*	m	3	346	Chopstick	?	?	?		R
1994	Takakuwa *et al.*	f	25	347	Ski pole			+		R
1994	Takakuwa *et al.*	m	9	347	Twig			+		L. via sinus maxillaris

1995	Bert *et al.*	m	52	274	Branch		+			R
1995	Fannin *et al.*	m	36	95	Display hook			+		R
1995	Hutchinson *et al.*	m	6	97	Clothes dryer		+			L
1995	Herman *et al.*	m	11	240	Pencil		+			R, not intracranial
1995	Herman *et al.*	f	3	240	Pencil		+?			L, not intracranial
1995	Kenigsberg *et al.*	m	3	308	Pencil		+			Perineum
1995	Sadiq and Thurairajan	m	10	107	Garden cane			+		L
1996	Miyagi *et al.*	m	4	290	Metal rod	?	?	?		L
1996	Potapov *et al.*	m	26	348	Piece of wood			+		R
1996	Rhatigan and Taylor	f	74	271	Pruned rose bush		+			R
1997	Kawamura *et al.*	m	4	192	Chopstick		+			L
1997	Lasky *et al.*	m	28	103	Pencil				+	R
1997	Lasky *et al.*	m	25	103	Toothbrush				+	R
1997	Seex *et al.*	f	71	26	Door key		+			R
1998	Kahler *et al.*	m	1	25	Fern		+			R
1998	Dinakaran and Noble	m	5	216	Pencil		+			R
1998	Matsumoto *et al.*	f	3	27	Chopstick		+			L
1998	Matsumoto *et al.*	m	57	27	Chopstick			+?		R
1998	Rao *et al.*	?	?	30	Spear	+?				R
1999	Smely	Infant	2	32	Twig		+			R
1999	Smely	m	35	32	Twig			+		R

* Same case as described by Oguz *et al.* in 1993 [164]

References

1. De Villiers JC, Sevel D. Intracranial complications of transorbital stab wounds. *Br J Ophthalmol.* 1975;59:52–56.
2. De Villiers JC. Stab wounds of brain and skull. In: Vinken OJ, Bruyn JW, eds. *Handbook of Clinical Neurology,* Vol 1. Amsterdam: North Holland Publ. Co. 1975:477–503. [Note: the revised series of this Handbook (1990) contained less information about TIPI.]
3. Hagan RE. Early complications following penetrating wounds of the brain. *J Neurosurg.* 1971;34:132–141.
4. Webster JE, Schneider RC, Lofstrom JE. Observations upon the management of orbito-cranial wounds. *J Neurosurg.* 1946;3:329–336.
5. Spoor TC. Penetrating orbital injuries. *Adv Ophthalmic Plastic Recontr Surg.* 1988;7:193–216.
6. Chapman PH, Grove AS. Early management of penetrating orbital injuries in children. *Conc Pediatr Neurosurg.* 1985;5:1–12.
7. Morrant Baker W. Perforating wounds of the orbit. *St Barth Hosp Rep.* 1888;24:179–196.
8. Duke-Elder S. Wounds of the adnexa: penetrating wounds of the orbit. In: Duke-Elder S, ed. *System of Ophthalmology,* Vol 14, Part 1. London: Kimpton. 1972:437–448.
9. Greig DM. Traversing wounds of the orbit. *Edinburgh Med J.* 1924;31: 241–262.
10. Kjer P. Orbital and transorbital stab wounds. *AMA Arch Ophthalmol.* 1954;51:811–821.
11. Wesley RE, Anderson SR, Weiss MR, Smith HP. Management of orbital–cranial trauma. *Adv Ophthalmic Plastic Reconstruct Surg.* 1988;7:3–26.
12. Bard LA, Jarrett WH. Intracranial complications of penetrating orbital injuries. *Arch Ophthalmol.* 1964;71:332–343.
13. Dujovny M, Manor RS, Israeli J. Orbitocranial foreign body. *Ophthalmologica.* 1974;168:261–268.
14. Courville CB, Schillinger RJ. Intracranial complications of diseases of eye and orbit. *Bull Los Angeles Neurolog Soc.* 1966;11:102–110.
15. Rowbotham GF. *Acute Injuries of the Head,* 3rd edn. Baltimore: Williams and Wilkins;1949:30–33.
16. McClure CC Jr, Gardner WJ. Transorbital intracranial stab wounds. *Cleveland Clin Q.* 1949;17:118–125.
17. Lavergne MG. Issue fatale rapide et imprévue d'une plaie perforante de l'orbite. *Bull Soc Belg Ophthalmol.* 1959;122:363–366.
18. Bursick DM, Selker RG. Intracranial pencil injuries. *Surg Neurol.* 1981;16: 427–431.

19. Wertheim S. Zur Kasuistik der durch die Orbita erfolgten Fremdkörperverletzungen des Gehirns. *Inaugural-Dissertation*, Giessen, 1904.
20. Coqueret MP. Contribution à l'étude des plaies pénétrantes du crane par la voie orbitaire. In: Steinheil G, ed. *Thèse de Paris.* Paris. 1905.
21. Verbiest H. Neurochirurgische aspecten van orbito-cranieële verwondingen in vredestijd. *Ned Tijdschr v Geneesk.* 1954;98:529–533.
22. De Grood MPAM, Goettsch FJB. Penetrating wound of the orbit. *Ophthalmologica.* 1958;135:159–160.
23. De Grood MPAM. *De indicatie tot de operatieve behandeling van de sacculaire aneurysmata in of nabij de circulus Willisii.* Proefschrift. 1966.
24. Copper A. Orbital cranial stab wounds. *Ophthalmologica.* 1957;134:366–372.
25. Kahler RJ, Tomlinson FH, Eisen DP, Masel JP. Orbitocranial penetration by a fern: Case report. *Neurosurgery.* 1998;42:1370–1373.
26. Seex K, Koppel D, Fitzpatrick M, Pyott A. Trans-orbital penetrating head injury with a door key. *J Cranio-Maxillofacial Surg.* 1997;25:353–355.
27. Matsumoto S, Hasuo K, Mizushima A *et al.* Intracranial penetrating injuries via the optic canal. *Am J Neuroradiol.* 1998;19:1163–1165.
28. Maya MM, Heier LA. Orbital CT, current use in the MR era. *Neuroimaging Clin N Am.* 1998;8:651–683.
29. McCabe MJ, Hammon WM, Halstead BW, Newton TH. A fatal brain injury caused by a needlefish. *Neuroradiology.* 1978;15:137–139.
30. Prakash Rao G, Rao NS, Reddy PK. Technique of removal of an impacted sharp object in a penetrating head injury using the lever principle. *Br J Neurosurg.* 1998;12:569–571.
31. Mains B, Nagle M. Thrombosis of the internal carotid artery due to soft palate injury. *J Laryngol Otol.* 1989;103:796–797.
32. Smely C, Orszagh M. Intracranial transorbital injury by a wooden foreign body: Re-evaluation of CT and MRI findings. *Br J Neurosurg.* 1999;13:206–211.
33. Scott J. Causes and observations illustrative of the fatal effect of puncture wounds of the orbit. *Edinburgh Med J.* 1834;43:359.
34. Faria MA Jr. The death of Henry II of France. *J Neurosurg.* 1992;77:964–969.
35. Betke D. Hirnabscess und Eiterige Meningitis nach Orbitalverletzung, mit eigenthümliche Verlauf. *Klin Mbl Augenhk.* 1869;7:182–186.
36. Editorial. *Lancet.* 1897;Jan 9:113–114.
37. Winkfield A. A case of compound fracture of the roof of the orbit; trephining; recovery. *Lancet.* 1897;Jan 2:38–39.
38. La Force. Plötzlichen Todesfall. *Schmidts Jahrbücher.* 1874;162:S174.
39. Adamük E. Zur Casuistik der Corpora aliena in der Orbita. *Klin Mbl Augenhk.* 1896;34:198–201.
40. Lotz A. Zwei Fälle von unerwartet grossen Fremdkörper der Orbita bei perforirenden Wangenverletzungen durch Sturz. *Klin Mbl Augenhk.* 1890;28: 365–370.
41. Annandale Th. Case in which a knitting-needle penetrated the brain through the orbit. *Edinburgh Med J.* 1877;126:891–894.
42. Pagenstecher H. Extraction eines fremden Körpers aus der Orbita und Schädelhöhle. *Klin Monatsbl Augenheilk.* 1864;166–171.
43. Dietz H. Über orbito-frontale perforierende Verletzungen. *Neurochirurgia.* 1980;23:219–223.

44. Polaillon. Perforation de la cavité orbitaire par l'extrémité d'une parapluie. *Bull Acad Méd Paris.* 1891;3e ser,26:192–193.
45. Laplace. Puncture through the orbit. *Lancet.* 1891;Dec 19th:1405–1406.
46. Ljunggren B. *Great Men with Sick Brains.* AANS. 1990:2–8.
47. Hoffman JR, Neuhaus RW, Bayliss HI. Penetrating orbital trauma. *Am J Emerg Med.* 1983;1:22–27.
48. du Trevou MD, van Dellen JR. Penetrating stabwounds to the brain: the timing of angiography in patients presenting with the weapon already removed. *Neurosurgery.* 1992;31:905–912.
49. Wuttke W. Phählungsverletzung des Gehirns bei einem Kleinkind. *Z Kinderheilk.* 1964;91:99–108.
50. Scarfo GB, Mariottini A, Palma L. Oculo-cerebral perforating trauma by foreign objects. *J Neurosurg Sci.* 1990;34:111–116.
52. Dunya IM, Rubin PA, Shore JW. Penetrating orbital trauma [review]. *Int Ophthalmol Clin.* 1995;35:25–36.
53. van Dellen JR, Lipschitz R. Stab wounds of the skull. *Surg Neurol.* 1978;10:110–114.
54. Herring CJ, Lumsden AB, Tindall SC. Transcranial stab wounds: a report of three cases and suggestions for management. *Neurosurgery.* 1988;23:658–662.
55. O'Neill OR, Gilliland G, Delashaw JB, Purtzer TJ. Transorbital penetrating head injury with a hunting arrow: case report. *Surg Neurol.* 1994;42:494–497.
56. Schneider RC, Henderson JW. Penetrating orbital wound with intracranial complications. *AMA Arch Ophthalmol.* 1952;47:81–85.
57. Dempsey LC, Winestock DP, Hoff JT. Stab wounds of the brain. *West J Med.* 1977;126:1–4.
57. Matson DD. Craniocerebral trauma in childhood. *Am J Surg.* 1961;101: 677–683.
58. Gouazé A, Santini JJ. Les traumatismes orbito-encéphaliques. *Neurochirurgie.* 1971;17:291–295.
59. Unger HH, Umbach W. Transorbitale Schädelhirntraumen durch Fremdkörper. *Klin Mbl Augenheilk.* 1963;140:269–281.
60. Michon J, Liu D. Intraorbital foreign bodies. *Semin Ophthalmol.* 1994;9:199.
61. Steavenson WE. An unusual case of hemiplegia. *St Barts Hosp Rep London.* 1879;15:287–289.
62. De Nobele J. Sur les plaies de l'orbite par pénétration des corps étrangers. *Flandre Med Grand.* 1895;2:129–137, 161–166.
63. Martial R. De l'hemiplégie traumatique. *Nouv Icon Salpêtr.* 1900;8:209–242.
64. Solieri S. Uber die Stichwunden des Gehirns von der Schädelbasis aus. *Arch Klin Chir.* 1914;105:153–169.
65. Nakayama M, Asakura T, Awa H, Atsugi M. Transorbital penetrating head injury – a case report. *Acta Med Univ Kagoshima.* 1986;28:29–36.
66. Kreft WW, Duffy JJ. Intra-orbital and intracranial foreign body. *Illinois Med J.* 1962;121:369–371.
67. Murphree HC, Broussard WJ. Pneumocephalus associated with injury of the orbit. *J Neurosurg.* 1965;23:450–451.
68. Viková E, Slapák I. Verletzungen der Augenhohle durch Fremdkörper. *Klin Mbl Augenheilk.* 1991;198:117–120.

69. Dabezies OH Jr, Naugle TC Sr, Naugle TC Jr. Penetrating orbital injury caused by an 'Afro comb'. *Ann Ophthalmol.* 1982;14:780–782.
70. Bramwell B. Case of left hemiplegia due to a perforating wound of the orbit. *Scot Med Surg J.* 1897;710.
71. Solomon KD, Pearson PA, Tetz MR, Baker RS. Cranial injury from unsuspected penetrating orbital trauma: a review of five cases. *J Trauma.* 1993;34:285–289.
72. Mansuy L, Rougier J, Fischer G. Corps étranger intra-orbitale et intra-cranien. *Bull Soc Ophthalmol Fr.* 1965;12:1127–1129.
73. De Villiers JC. Sixteen cases of transorbital stabwounds of the head. *J Neurol Neurosurg Psychiatr.* 1975;38:822.
74. Michon JJ, Miller NR. Management of combined penetrating intraorbital and intracranial trauma. *Arch Ophthalmol.* 1993;111:438–439.
75. Mono J, Hollenberg RD, Harvey JT. Occult transorbital intracranial penetrating injuries. *Ann Emerg Med.* 1986;15:589–591.
76. Svoboda J. An injury of the orbit and the base of the skull with fatal termination. *Ceskoslov Oftal.* 1948;4:72–74. [Abstract in *Ophthalmol Lit.* 1948;2:422.]
77. Specht CS, Varga JH, Jalali MM, Edelstein JP. Orbitocranial wooden foreign body diagnosed by magnetic resonance imaging. *Surv Ophthalmol.* 1992;36: 341–344.
78. Guthkelch AN. Apparently trivial wounds of the eyelids with intracranial damage. *Br Med J.* 1960;2:842–844.
79. Yamamoto I, Yamada S, Sato O. Unusual craniocerebral penetrating injury by a chopstick. *Surg Neurol.* 1985;23:396–398.
80. Yamashita T, Kadota K, Asakura T, Ohba N. Penetrating orbitocranial injury. Report of a case by chopstick. *Orbit.* 1988;7:59–64.
81. Amano K, Kamano S. Cerebellar abscess due to penetrating orbital wound. *J Comput Assist Tomogr.* 1982;6:1163–1166.
82. Rahimizadeh A, Shakeri M, Amirdjamshidi A. Unusual craniocerebral injuries by glass fragments. *Neurosurgery.* 1987;21:437–438.
83. Vander JF, Nelson CC. Penetrating orbital injury with cavernous sinus involvement. *Ophthalmic Surg.* 1988;19:328–330.
84. Haase A. Phälungsverletzung des Gehirns durch die Orbita mit tödlichem Ausgang. *Z Augenheilk.* 1929;69:230–237.
85. Gatchell HV. Foreign body removed from the orbit. *Br Med J.* 1923;1:283.
86. Le Win Th. Tea spoon penetrating child's orbit. *Arch Ophthalmol.* 1952;47: 515.
87. Palin AG. A case in the west of England. *Trans Ophthalmol Soc UK.* 1948;68:351.
88. Klug N. Penetrating orbito-cranial injuries. *Mod Asp Neurosurg Excerpta Med.* 1973;4:75–80.
89. Lawson D, Glastonbury J, Oatey P. An unusual intracerebral foreign body associated with eye trauma. *Austr NZ J Ophthalmol.* 1990;18:221–223.
90. Bank DE, Carolan PL. Cerebral abscess formation following ocular trauma: A hazard associated with common wooden toys. *Pediatr Emerg Care.* 1993;9:285–288.
91. Baron P. An unusual cause of penetrating exophthalmos. *Br J Surg.* 1937; 25:459–460.

92. Noterman J, Rétif J, Klastersky J. Staphylococcal meningitis and abscess associated with intracranial foreign body, as a late complication of cranial trauma. *Acta Neurochir.* 1973;29:131–136.
93. Anderson RL, Carroll TF, Harvey JT, Myers MG. Petriellidum (allescheria) boydii orbital and brain abscess treated with intravenous miconazole. *Am J Ophthalmol.* 1984;97:771–775.
94. Papadopoulos M, McCurrach F, Carlisle I. Orbital impalement by steering wheel lock. *Austr NZ J Ophthalmol.* 1994;22:278–279.
95. Fannin LA, Fitch CP, Raymond WR, Flanagan JC, Mazzoli RA. Eye injuries from merchandise display hooks. *Am J Ophthalmol.* 1995;120:397–399.
96. Walchshofer E. Über eine Stichverletzung, die durch die rechte Orbita in das Schädelinnere drang. *Dtsch Zeitschr Chirurg.* 1928;209:397–400.
97. Hutchison BM, Webb LA, Pyott AA, Barrie T. Penetrating orbitocranial trauma in the absence of an externally visible entry wound. *Orbit.* 1995;14:53–56.
98. Kane N, Jamjoon A, Teimory M. Penetrating orbitocranial injury. *Injury.* 1991;22:326–327.
99. Beauchamp JO, Miller GR. Unusual orbital foreign body. *Am J Ophthalmol.* 1967;63:868.
100. Little WS. Case of fatal injury to the brain. *Dublin Q J Med Sci.* 1851;12:226.
101. Jamieson P. Case of fatal injury to the orbit with a walking stick. *Month J Med Sci Edinburgh.* 1855;20:514.
102. Thomson JR, Harwood-Nash DC, Fitz CR. Cerebral aneurysm in children. *Am J Roentgenol.* 1973;118:163–175.
103. Lasky JB, Epley D, Karesh JW. Household objects as a cause of self-inflicted orbital apex syndrome. *J Trauma.* 1997;42:555–558.
104. Guttierrez A, Gil L, Sahuquillo J, Rubio E. Unusual penetrating craniocerebral injury. *Surg Neurol.* 1983;19:541–543.
105. Windle-Taylor PC. Transorbital injury from a harpoon involving the paranasal sinuses. *ORL.* 1978;40:278–284.
106. Wesly RE, McCord CD. Tension pneumocephalus from orbital roof fracture. *Ann Ophthalmol.* 1982;14:184–190.
107. Sadiq SA, Thurairajan G. A case of transorbital intracranial damage underlying a seemingly innocuous injury. *Injury.* 1995;26:279–280.
108. Miller CF, Brodkey JS, Colombi BJ. The danger of intracranial wood. *Surg Neurol.* 1977;7:95–103.
109. Meritt RD, Chisholm L, Ross Fleming AF, Schwartz ML. Foreign body penetration through the superior orbital fissure. *Arch Ophthalmol.* 1973;90:67–68.
110. Birch-Hirschfeld A. Die Stichverletzungen der Orbita. In: Graefe A, Saemisch T, eds. *Handbuch der Gesamte Augenheilkunde.* Berlin: Springer Verlag. 1930;9:998–1004.
111. Morrissey ThB, Byrd CR, Deitch EA. The incidence of recurrent penetrating trauma in an urban trauma center. *J Trauma.* 1991;31:1536–1538.
112. Tomita T, Miwa T. Penetrating cranio-cerebral injuries in childhood. Report of three cases. *Nerv Syst Child.* 1987;3:229–234.
113. Sarda RP, Sharma RG, Ratnawat PS. Deep perforating injury of the orbit. *Eye Ear Nose Throat Monogr.* 1970;49:44–46.
114. Agarwal PK, Kumar H, Srivastava PK. Unusual orbital foreign bodies. *Ind J Ophthalmol.* 1993;41:125–127.

115. Sedan J, Paillas JE. Tige métallique de six centimètres intra-orbito-cranienne. *Rev Oto'-Neuro-Ophthalmol.* 1953;25:401–405.
116. Duffy GP, Bandari YS. Intracranial complications following transorbital penetrating injuries. *Br J Surg.* 1969;56:685–688.
117. Prideaux E. Penetrating wound of the orbit involving the brain. *Lancet.* 1882;2:846.
118. Takvam JA, Midelfart A. Survey of eye injuries in Norwegian children. *Acta Ophthalmol. (Copenhagen).* 1993;71:500–505.
119. Sollmann WP, Seifert V, Haubitz B, Dietz H. Combined orbito-frontal injuries. *Neurosurg Rev.* 1989;12:115–121.
120. Winckler G. Anatomie de l'orbite et ses rapports avec les cavités voisines. *Confin Neurol.* 1966;28:165–173.
121. Lagrange F. The orbital cavity. *Adv Ophthalmol Plastic Reconstr Surg.* 1987;6:7–16.
122. Lubeck D. Penetrating ocular injuries. *Emerg Med Clin N Am.* 1988;6: 127–146.
123. Simonton JT, Arthurs BP. Penetrating injuries to the orbit. *Adv Ophthalmic Plastic Recontr Surg.* 1988;7:217–227.
124. Wolfe SA. The orbit – cone or pyramid? [letter]. *Ann Plast Surg.* 1980;5:340.
125. Weisman RA. Surgical anatomy of the orbit. *Otolaryngol Clin N Am.* 1988; 21:1–12.
126. Asbury CC, Castillo M, Mukherji SK. Review of computed tomographic imaging in acute orbital trauma. *Emerg Radiol.* 1995;2:367–375.
127. Flanagan JC, McLachlan DL, Shannon GM. Orbital roof fractures: Neurologic and neurosurgical considerations. *Ophthalmology.* 1980;87:325–329.
128. Swanson JL, Augustine JA. Penetrating intracerebral trauma from a fishhook. *Ann Emerg Med.* 1992;21:568–571.
129. Scharf J, Zonis S. Proptosis as a presenting symptom of orbital foreign body. *J Pediatr Ophthalmol.* 1977;14:176–177.
130. Anavi Y, Calderon S. Metallic foreign body in the orbit. *Ann Ophthalmol.* 1994;26:17–19.
131. Dogliotti AM. Technique et indications de la ventriculographie cérébrale par la voie transvoute-orbitaire. *Bull Memb Soc Natl Chir.* 1934; Seance 11: Tome LX, No. 25.
132. Fiamberti AM. Proposta di una technica operatoria modificata e simplificata per gli interventi all Moniz sui lobi prefrontali in malati di mente. *Rass Studi Psichiatr.* 1937;26:797–803.
133. Freeman W. Transorbital leucotomy. *Lancet.* 1948;2:371–373.
134. Teng MMH, Lirng JF, Chang T *et al.* Embolization of carotid cavernous fistula by means of direct puncture through the superior orbital fissure. *Radiology.* 1995;194:705–711.
135. Ehlers H. The orbit—a survey. *Acta Ophthalmol (Copenhagen).* 1970;48: 571–577.
136. Dimitrakopoulos I, Lazaridis N, Karakasis D. Unusual retained foreign body in the orbit. *J Oral Maxillofac Surg.* 1991;49:420–421.
137. Duke-Elder S. *Textbook of Ophthalmology,* Vol 6, *Injuries.* St Louis CV: Mosby. 1954:6313–6325.

138. Teng MMH, Guo WY, Lee LS, Chang T. Direct puncture of the cavernous sinus for the obliteration of a recurrent carotid–cavernous fistula. *Neurosurgery.* 1988;23:104–107.
139. Lee KF, Lin S. Unusual penetrating injury of the orbit. *Am J Roentgenol.* 1971;122:349–351.
140. Gates TR, Hardjasudarma M. Computed tomography findings of an intraorbital pencil [letter]. *Am J Emerg Med.* 1993;11:433–434.
141. Youngshu C, Guojun Z. Transorbital cranial injuries caused by chopstick and glass splinters. *Chin Med J.* 1980;93:487–490.
142. Heyworth P, Kon C, Tabandeh H. Unsuspected orbitocranial injury following ocular trauma. *Br J Hosp Medicine* 1994;51:174–175.
143. Rao RM, Sekhar NC, Daniel SM. Retained foreign body in orbit with intracranial extension. *Ind J Ophthalmol.* 1993;41:86–87.
144. Gottlieb RD, Meitelesh Z, Liebeskind AL, Kimmelman CP. Foreign body of the skull base due to transorbital penetrating trauma. *Otolaryngol Head Neck Surg.* 1992;107(6 Pt.1):800–802.
145. Shriwas SR, Kinzha AZ. Orbital injuries in children: play-related. *Ind J Ophthalmol.* 1993;41:129–130.
146. Hansen JE, Gudeman SK, Holgate RC, Saunders RA. Penetrating intracranial wood wounds: clinical limitations of computerized tomography. *J Neurosurg.* 1988;68:752–756.
147. Irwin GE, Tilelli J. Unrecognized penetrating intracranial foreign body. *Am J Emerg Med.* 1986;4:412–413.
148. Coro CM, Thiede C, Podlesh S. Pencil injury. *Oral Surg Oral Med Pathol.* 1993;76:256.
149. Jackson FE, Schonder AA, Cook RC, Wilcox JR, Whitely RH. Transorbital, transcranial stab wound. *JAMA.* 1971;215:1649–1651.
150. Colley T. Penetrating wounds of the orbit. *Br J Ophthalmol.* 1934;18:241–251.
151. Weisman RA, Savino PJ, Schut L, Schatz NJ. Computed tomography in penetrating wounds of the orbit with retained foreign bodies. *Arch Otolaryngol.* 1983;109:265–268.
152. Mutlukan E, Fleck BW, Cullen JF, Whittle IR. Case of penetrating orbitocranial injury caused by wood. *Br J Ophthalmol.* 1991;75:374–376.
153. Yamaguchi T, Hata H, Hiratsuka H, Suganuma Y, Inaba Y. [Penetrating transorbital brain injury and intracranial foreign body.] *No Shinkei Geka.* 1978;6:183–184.
154. Kala M, Houdek M, Andrs M. Unusual penetrating craniocerebral injury. *Acta Univ Palacki Olomuc Fac Med.* 1989;121:341–344.
155. Schmidt JGH, Frowein RA. Orbito-kraniobasale Pfählungsverletzungen. *Klin Monatsbl Augenheilk.* 1971;159:624–632.
156. Siegel EB, Bastek JV, Mehringer CM, Yee RD. Fatal intracranial extension of an orbital umbrella stab injury. *Ann Ophthalmol.* 1983;15:99–102.
157. Zentner J, Hassler W, Petersen D. A wooden foreign body penetrating the superior orbital fissure. *Neurochirurgia.* 1991;34:188–190.
158. Gonçalves da Silva CE, Gonçalves de Silva JA. Eine seltene orbito-zerebrale Messerstichverletzung. *Neurochirurgia.* 1979;22:28–30.
159. McEwen CJ, Fullarton G. A penetrating orbitocranial stab wound. *Br J Ophthalmol.* 1986;70:147–149.

160. Oguz M, Aksungur EH, Atilla E, Altay M, Soyupak SK, Ildan F. Orbitocranial penetration of a pencil: extraction under CT control. *Eur J Radiol.* 1993;17:85–87.
161. Albert DM, Burns WP, Scheie HG. Severe orbitocranial foreign-body injury. *Am J Ophthalmol.* 1965;60:1109.
162. Mohssenipour I, Twerdy K. Ein Beitrag zu den Stichverletzungen des Gehirns. *Wien Klin Wochenschr.* 1977;89:551–553.
163. Gossman HH. Penetrating wound of the orbit. *Br Med J.* 1967;839–840.
164. Kessler L. Beitrag zur Pfälungsverletzung des Gehirns. *Dtsch Ges Wesen.* 1972;27:2441–2442.
165. Kupusarevic S. [Penetrating injuries of the orbit with report on an unusual case.] English abstract. *Med Pregl.* 1977;30:47–50.
166. Ho VT, McGuckin JF Jr, Smergel EM. Intraorbital wooden foreign body: CT and MR appearance. *AJNR Am J Neuroradiol.* 1996;17:134–136.
167. Hickman DM. Benign sequelae of a transorbital stabwound: an usual case report. *Ann Plast Surg.* 1984;12:279–283.
168. Field HB. Foreign body (curtain rod) penetrating orbit, pharynx and neck, with complete recovery. *AMA Arch Ophthalmol.* 1951;46:157–158.
169. Henry RC. Infra-orbital penetrating foreign body. *J Laryngol Otol.* 1972;86: 1159–1162.
170. Freiwald MJ. Penetrating wound of the orbit: a 31 year follow-up. *Br J Ophthalmol.* 1977;61:544–546.
171. Horner FA, Berry RG, Frantz M. Broken pencil points as a cause of brain abscess. *N Eng J Med.* 1964;271:342–345.
172. Mezue WC, Saddeqi N, Ude A. Barbed spear to the skull base: case report. *Neurosurgery.* 1991;28:428–430.
173. Flieringa HJ. Orbita fistels. *Ned Tijdschr v Geneesk.* 1950;94:1163.
174. Rahman NU, Jamjoon A, Jamjoon ZA, Abu el-Asrar. An orbital–cranial injury caused by penetrating metallic foreign bodies: report of two cases. *Int Ophthalmol.* 1997;21:13–17.
175. de Tribolet N, Guignard G, Zander E. Brain abscess after transnasal intracranial penetration of a paint-brush. *Surg Neurol.* 1979;11:187–189.
176. Davis EDD. Abscess in frontal lobe of brain. *Proc R Soc Med.* 1934;27: 1285–1288.
177. Tokitsu M, Nakamura M, Yokoyama H, Watanabe H, Hara M, Takeuchi K. [Skullbase-penetrating injuries caused by umbrella tips: case reports.] English abstract. *No Shinkei Geka.* 1990;18:189–192.
178. Fallon MJ, Plante DM, Brown LW. Wooden transnasal intracranial penetration: an unusual presentation. *J Emerg Med.* 1992;10:439–443.
179. Inbasekaran V, Jawahar G, Natarajan M. Brain abscess caused by pencil tip injury. *J Ind Med Assoc.* 1985;83:284.
180. Healy JF. Computed tomography of a cranial wooden foreign body. *J Comput Assist Tomogr.* 1980;4:555–556.
181. Udwadia RA, Maniar D, Acharya M. A transethmoid transorbital foreign body. *J Laryngol Otol.* 1994;108:441–442.
182. Levin LA, Joseph MP. Penetrating trauma with a meat thermometer. *J Trauma.* 1996;41:926–929.

183. Mirza GE, Ekinciler OF, Karaküçük S. Diagnosis and management of a biorbital pencil injury. *Acta Ophthalmolog.* 1992;70:266–269.
184. Quayle AA. The significance of small wounds of the eyelids. *Br J Oral Maxillofac Surg.* 1986;24:17–21.
185. Hungerford J. A penetrating orbitocranial injury presenting as a gaze palsy [letter]. *J Neurol Neurosurg Psychiatr.* 1982;45:1072–1073.
186. Medler A. Holzkeilverletzung von Orbita, mittlerer und hinterer Schädelgrube mit überraschend geringer Verletzungsfolgen. *Mbl Augenhk.* 1956;129: 543–546.
187. Sebag J, Shillito J, Robb R. Transorbital penetrating injuries to the frontal lobe. *Ophthalmic Surg.* 1968;17:631–634.
188. Aichmair H. Orbital impalement injury. An unusual case. *Trans Ophthalmol Soc UK.* 1980;100:483–484.
189. Vérin Ph, Vildy A, Benjelloun D. Méningite par traumatisme orbitaire. *Bull Soc Ophthal Fr.* 1976;76:969–970.
190. McCaughey AD. An unusual infra-orbital foreign body. *Br J Oral Maxillofac Surg.* 1988;26:426–429.
191. Vandertop WP, Vries WB, Swieten J, Tamos LMP. Recurrent brain abscess due to an unexpected foreign body. *Surg Neurol.* 1992;37:39–41.
192. Kawamura S, Hadeishi H, Sasaguchi N, Suzuki A, Yasui N. Penetrating head injury caused by chopstick. Case report. *Neurol Medico-Chirurgica.* 1997; 37:332–335.
193. Doucet TW, Harper DW, Rogers J. Penetrating orbital foreign body with intracranial involvement. *Ann Ophthalmol.* 1983;15:325–327.
194. Bullock R, van Dellen JR. Acute carotid–cavernous fistula with retained knife blade after transorbital stab wound. *Surg Neurol.* 1985;24:555–558.
195. Ide CH, Webb RW. Penetrating transorbital injury with cerebrospinal orbitorrhea. *Am J Ophthalmol.* 1971;71:1037–1039.
196. Stewart DJ, Polomeno RC. Total transient visual loss and orbital foreign bodies. *Can J Ophthal.* 1979;14:95–98.
197. Larmande A, Descuns P, Margaillan A. Plaie d l'orbite avec hémiplégie homolatérale chez un escrimeur. *Rev d'Oto-neuro-ophthal.* 1956;28:440–441.
198. Goald HJ, Ronderos A. Traumatic perforation of the intracranial portion of the internal carotid artery with eleven-day survival. *J Neurosurg.* 1961;18: 401–404.
199. Nuel JP. Paralysie du nerf oculomoteur externe comme seul symptôme d'une déchirure traumatique de l'artère carotide interne dans le sinus caverneux. *Soc Belge Ophthalmol (Brux).* 1901;30–45.
200. Decroix G, Pendriel G. Paralysie du nerf moteur oculaire commun consécutive à la pénétration orbito-crânienne d'une antenne métallique. *Bull Soc Ophthalmol Fr.* 1974;12:1137–1141.
201. Castelain, Lafargue. Du tétanos consécutif aux lésions oculaires. *Ann Ocul.* 1920;157:9–26.
202. Bullock MH, Baker GS, Henderson JW. Injuries of brain caused by penetration of the orbit. *Minnesota Med.* 1959;42:1408–1413.
203. Cartwright MJ, Kurumety UR, Frueh BR. Intraorbital wood foreign body. *Ophthalmic Plastic Reconstr Surg.* 1995;11:44–48.

204. Tate E, Cupples H. Detection of orbital foreign bodies with computed tomography: current limits. *Am J Roentgenol.* 1981;137:493–495.
205. Ossoinig KC. Detection of wood foreign bodies. Authors' reply (Green BF, Kraft SP). *Ophthalmology.* 1991;98:274–275.
206. Neubaur H, Frowein RA, Schmidt JGH, Ruessmann W. Intra-orbital foreign bodies. *Mod Probl Ophthal.* 1975;14:482–488.
207. Jacobson JA, Powell A, Craig JG, Bouffard JA, van Holsbeeck MT. Wooden foreign bodies in soft tissue: detection at US. *Radiology.* 1998;206:45–48.
208. Kazarian EL, Stokes NA, Flynn JT. The orbital puncture wound: intracranial complications of a retained foreign body. *J Paediatr Ophthalmol Strabismus.* 1980;17:247.
209. Charteris DG. Posterior penetrating injury of the orbit with retained foreign body. *Br J Ophthalmol.* 1988;72:432–433.
210. Patten JT. Penetrating transorbital foreign body with ocular preservation. *Ann Ophthalmol.* 1975;7:651–654.
211. Waring GO III, Flanagan JC. Pneumocephalus: A sign of intracranial involvement in orbital fractures. *Arch Ophthalmol.* 1975;93:847–850.
212. Trommer G, Kösling S, Nerkelun S, Gosch D, Klöppel R. Darstellbarkeit von Orbita – Fremdkörpern in der CT. Ist die Fremdkörperübersicht noch sinnvoll? *Fortschr Röntgenstr.* 1997;166:487–492.
213. Lunsford LD, Woodford J, Drayer BP. Cranial computed tomographic demonstration of intracranial penetration by an orbital foreign body. *Neurosurgery.* 1977;1:57–59.
214. Osborn AG, Daines JH, Wing SD, Anderson RE. Intracranial air on computed tomography. *J Neurosurg.* 1978;48:355–359.
215. McHugh D, Mosely RP, Uttley D. Clostridium perfringes brain infection following a penetrating wound to the orbit. *J Neurol Neurosurg Psychiatr.* 1987;50:241.
216. Dinakaran S, Noble PJ. Silent orbitocranial penetration by a pencil. *J Accid Emerg Med.* 1998;15:274–275.
217. Mikhael MA, Mattar AG. Case report: chronic graphite granulomatous abscess simulating a brain tumor. *J Comput Assist Tomogr.* 1997;1:513–516.
218. Lydiatt DD, Hollins RR, Moyer DJ, Davis LF. Problems in evaluation of penetrating foreign bodies with computed tomography scans. *J Oral Maxillofac Surg.* 1987;45:965–968.
219. Grove AS. Orbital trauma and computed tomography. *Ophthalmology.* 1980;87:403–411.
220. Roberts CF, Leehey PJ. Intraorbital wood foreign body mimicking air at CT. *Radiology.* 1992;185:507–508.
221. Ginsberg LE, Williams DW III, Mathews VP. CT in penetrating craniocervical injury by wooden foreign bodies: reminder of a pitfall. *Am J Neuroradiol.* 1992;14:892–895.
222. Lustrin ES, Brown JH, Noveline R, Weber AL. Radiologic assessment of trauma and foreign bodies of the eye and the orbit. *Neuroimaging Clin N Am.* 1996;6:219–237.
223. Pyhtinen J, Ilkko E, Lähde S. Wooden foreign bodies in CT. Case reports and experimental studies. *Acta Radiol.* 1995;36:148–151.

224. McGuckin JF Jr, Akhtar N, Ho VT, Smergel EM, Kubacki EJ, Villafana T. CT and MR evaluation of a wooden foreign body in an *in vitro* model of the orbit. *AJNR Am J Neuroradiol.* 1996;17:129–133.
225. Kadir S, Aronow S, David KR. The use of computer tomography in the detection of intraorbital foreign bodies. *Comput Tomogr.* 1977;1:151–156.
226. Jooma R, Bradshaw JR, Coakham HB. Computed tomography in penetrating cranial injury by a wooden foreign body. *Surg Neurol.* 1984;21:236–238.
227. Myllylä V, Pyhtinen J, Päivänsalo M, Tervonen O, Koskela P. CT detection and localisation of intraorbital foreign bodies: experiments with wood and glass. *Fortsch Röntgenstr.* 1987;146:639–643.
228. Gückel C. Computertomographische und kernspintomographische Nachweismöglichkeit hölzerner Fremdkörper nach perforierender Augenverletzung. *Radiologe.* 1988;28:334–337.
229. Glatt HJ, Custer PL, Barrett L, Sartor K. Magnetic resonance imaging and computed tomography in a model of wooden foreign bodies in the orbit. *Ophthalmol Plast Reconstr Surg.* 1990;6:108–114.
230. Wesly RE, Wahl JW, Loden JP, Henderson RR. Management of wooden foreign bodies in the orbit. *South Med J.* 1982;75:924–926.
231. Saini JS, Mohan K, Khandalavala B. Wooden foreign bodies of the orbit. A diagnostic dilemma. *Orbit.* 1989;8:139–142.
232. Green BF, Kraft SP, Carter KD, Buncic JR, Nerad JA, Armstrong D. Intraorbital wood: detection by magnetic resonance imaging. *Ophthalmology.* 1990;97: 608–611.
233. Dalley RW. Intraorbital wood foreign bodies on CT: use of wide bone window settings to distinguish wood from air. *Am J Roentgenol.* 1995;164:434–435.
234. Braun J, Gdal-on M, Goldsher D, Borovich B, Guilburd JN. Traumatic carotid aneurysm secondary to cavernous sinus penetrating by wood; CT features. *J Comput Assist Tomogr.* 1987;11:525–528.
235. Kuhns LR, Borlaza GS, Seigel RS, Paramagul CH, Berger PE. An *in vitro* comparison of computed tomography, xeroradiography, and radiography in the detection of soft-tissue foreign bodies. *Radiology.* 1979;132:218–219.
236. Lindahl S. Computed tomography of intra orbital foreign bodies. *Acta Radiol.* 1987;28:235–240.
237. Macrae JA. Diagnosis and management of a wooden orbital foreign body: case report. *Br J Ophthalmol.* 1979;63:848–851.
238. Kaiser MC, Rodesch G, Capesius P. CT in a case of intracranial penetration of a pencil. *Neuroradiology.* 1983;24:229–231.
239. Woolfson JM, Wesley RE. Magnetic resonance imaging and computed tomographic scanning of fresh (green) wood foreign bodies in dog orbits. *Ophthalmol Plast Reconstr Surg.* 1990;6:237–240.
240. Herman TE, Shackelford GD, Tychsen L. Unrecognized retention of intraorbital graphite pencil fragments: the role of computerized tomography. *Pediatr Radiol.* 1995;25:535–537.
241. Nelson EW, DeHart MM, Christensen AW, Smith DK. Magnetic resonance imaging characteristics of a lead pencil foreign body in the hand. *J Hand Surg [AM].* 1996;21:100–103.
242. Wilson WB, Dreisbach JN, Lattin DE, Stears JC. Magnetic resonance imaging of nonmetallic orbital foreign bodies. *Am J Ophthalmol.* 1988;105:612–617.

243. Kulshrestha M, Misson G. Magnetic resonance imaging and the dangers of orbital foreign bodies [letter]. *Br J Ophthalmol.* 1995;1149.
244. Kelly WM, Paglen PG, Pearson JA, San Diego AG, Solomon MA. Ferromagnetism of intraocular foreign body causes unilateral blindness after MR study. *AJNP.* 1986;7:243–245.
245. Kieck CF, De Villiers JC. Vascular lesions due to transcranial stab wounds. *J Neurosurg.* 1984;60:42–46.
246. Girouard Y, Delage G, Mathieu JP, Larbrisseau A. Meningitis and brain abscess due to clostridium perfringes and clostridium paraputrificum following orbital trauma. *Can J Neurol Sci.* 1981;8:309–311.
247. Cressman MR, Hayes GJ. Traumatic aneurysm of the anterior choroidal artery. *J Neurosurg.* 1966;24:102–104.
248. Bakay L, Glausauer FE, Grand W. Unusual intracranial foreign bodies. *Acta Neurochir (Wien).* 1977;39:219–231.
249. Devi BI, Bhatia S, Kak VK. Penetrating orbito-cranial injuries. Report of two cases. *Ind J Ophthalmol.* 1993;41:84–86.
250. Ferry DJ Jr, Kempe LG. False aneurysm secondary to penetration of the brain through orbitofacial wounds. *J Neurosurg.* 1972;36:503–506.
251. Carothers A. Orbitofacial wounds and cerebral artery injuries caused by umbrella tips. *JAMA.* 1978;239:1151–1152.
252. Fein W, Carton ChA. Transorbital removal of intracranial foreign body in middle fossa. *Ann Ophthalmol.* 1976;8:89–92.
253. Carver GM Jr, Durham NC, Patterson W. Transorbital cranial foreign body. *Surgery.* 1954;35:475–481.
254. Fanning WL, Willett LR, Phillips CF, Wallman LJ. Puncture wound of the eyelid causing brain abscess. *J Trauma.* 1976;16:919–920.
255. Verbiest H. Post-traumatic pulsating exophthalmus. *J Neurosurg.* 1953;10: 264–271.
256. Haszler W, Eggert HR. Extradural and intradural microsurgical approaches to lesions of the optic canal and the superior orbital fissure. *Acta Neurochir.* 1985;74:87–93.
257. Baba M, Tachizawa T, Takizawa H, Sugiara, K. [Penetrating transorbital intracranial foreign body.] English abstract. *No Shinkei Geka.* 1982;10: 869–874.
258. Dujovny M, Osgood CP, Maroon JC, Janetta PJ. Penetrating intracranial foreign bodies in children. *J Trauma.* 1975;15:981–986.
259. Greene KA, Zabramski JM. Orbital and intracranial injury in a 7-year-old boy [letter; comment]. *J Trauma.* 1994;37:513–514.
260. Kasamo S, Asakura T, Kusomoto K, Nakayama M, Kadota K, Atsuchi M, Yamamoto Y. [Transorbital penetrating brain injury.] English abstract. *No Shinkei Geka.* 1992;20:433–438.
261. Ildan F, Bagdatoglu H, Boyar B, Doganay M, Cetinalp E, Karadayi A. The nonsurgical treatment of penetrating orbito-cranial injury. *J Trauma.* 1994;36: 116–118.
262. Klimek L, Laborde G, Mösges R, Wenzel M. Ein neues Verfahren zur Entfernung von Fremkörper in Kofpbereich. *Unfallchirurg.* 1993;96:213–216.
263. Ersahin Y, Mutluer S, Güzelbag E. Transorbital stab wound: a case report. *Turk J Pediatr.* 1994;36:71–75.

264. Greene KA, Dickman CA, Smith KA, Kinder EJ, Zabramski JM. Self-inflicted orbital and intracranial injury with a retained foreign body. *Surg Neurol.* 1993;40:499–503.
265. Nath FP, Teasdale E, Mendelow AD. Penetrating injury of the tuberculum sellae. *Neurosurgery.* 1984;14:598–600.
266. Klug W, Tzonos T. Über zwei, durch grosse Transorbital eingedrungene Fremdkörper verursachte Hirnverletzungen. *Zbl Neurochir.* 1961;21:56–61.
267. Stöwsand D. Transorbital Messerstichverletzung der linken Groszhirn-Hemisphäre und ihre neurologische Kompensation. *Zbl Neurochir.* 1967;28: 317–322.
268. Klotz F. Pencil penetrates orbit. *Am J Ophthalmol.* 1948;31:1636.
269. Stadler HE, Manders K, Marks J, Bonsett CH. Recurrent (bilocular?) brain abscess due to unusual foreign body – a case report. *J Indiana State Med Assoc.* 1973;65:799–802.
270. Foy P, Sharr M. Cerebral abscesses in children after pencil-tip injuries. *Lancet.* 1980;662–663.
271. Rhatigan MC, Taylor RH. A potentially life-threatening upper eyelid laceration. *Injury.* 1996;27:229–230.
272. Platt ES. Orbito-cranial penetrating injuries. *Am J Ophthalmol.* 1954;37: 758–763.
273. Coogan P, DeBehbke D. Occult penetrating orbital trauma. *Am J Emerg Med.* 1993;11:396–399.
274. Bert F, Ouahes O, Lambert-Zechovsky N. Brain abscess due to Bacillus macerans following a penetrating orbital injury. *J Clin Microbiol.* 1995;33: 1950–1953.
275. Jones BL, Hanson MF, Logan NA. Isolation of Bacillus licheniformis from a brain abscess following a penetrating orbital injury [letter]. *J Infect.* 1992;24: 103–104.
276. Sullivan TJ, Patel BC, Aylward GW, Wright JE. Anaerobic orbital abscess secondary to intraorbital wood. *Aust NZ J Ophthalmol.* 1993;21:49–52.
277. Shima T, Uozumi T, Nishimura S, Nishida M, Tao S. [False traumatic aneurysm secondary to penetration of the brain through supraorbital wound – report of a case]. English abstract. *No Shinkei Geka.* 1978;6:1025–1030.
278. Bullier B, Maisongrosse G, Mohieddine M, Millet P. Plaie pénétrante de l'orbite par baleine de parapluie avec ophthalmoplégie. *Bull Soc Ophthalmol Fr.* 1976;76:549–551.
279. Baldauf F. Traumatischer Hirnabcess mit 40 jähriger Latenzzeit. *Mschr Unfallheilk.* 1962;65:358–360.
280. Pilcher C. Penetrating wounds of the brain: an experimental study. *Ann Surg.* 1936;103:173–198.
281. Muscas M. Su due particolari casi di meningite emorragica da ferita dell'orbita. *Bull Oculist.* 1952;31:703–706.
282. Blumberg J, Johnston E. The forensic pathologist and unsuspected foreign body. *Forensic Sci.* 1963;8:231–249.
283. Slaughter H, Alvis BY. Pneumoencephalocele secondary to puncture wound of the lid. *Am J Ophthalmol.* 1944;27:617–620.
284. Bard LA. Pneumocephalus secondary to penetrating orbital wound. *Arch Ophthalmol.* 1963;70:232–235.

285. Markham JW. The clinical features of pneumocephalus based on a survey of 284 cases with report of 11 additional cases. *Acta Neuroch.* 1967;16:1–78.
286. Shevach I, Manor RS, Rappaport ZH. Orbital porencephalic cyst following penetrating orbitocranial trauma. *Childs Nerv Syst.* 1992;8:297–299.
287. Heyner FJ, Passmore JW. Pseudotumor of orbit. *Am J Ophthalmol.* 1965;59: 490–492.
288. Ferguson EC. Deep wooden foreign bodies of the orbit. A report of two cases. *Trans Am Acad Ophthalmol.* 1970;74:778–787.
289. Freitas MAL, Filho CAB, Lima R, Marchiori E. Traumatic ophthalmic fistula simulating carotid-cavernous fistula. *Neurosurgery.* 1983;12:102–104.
290. Miyagi A, Maeda K, Sugawara T. [Intraorbital conjunctival cyst after perforating orbital injury: a case report.] English abstract. *No Shinkei Geka.* 1996;24: 649–653.
291. Hsu CHY, Wang SJ. CSF leakage into the orbit demonstrated by Tc-99m DTPA cisternography. *Clin Nucl Med.* 1994;19:463.
292. Nagahiro S, Kaku M, Matsukado Y, Ogawa H, Kosaka H, Wada H. Penetrating craniocerebral injuries. *Neurol Surg (Tokyo).* 1981;9:1313–1318.
293. Walsh L, Hoyt W. Carotid cavernous fistula due to a stab wound. In: *Clinical Neuro-ophthalmology,* 3rd edn, Vol 2. Baltimore: Williamson and Wilkins. 1969:1714.
294. Khalil N, Elwany MN, Miller JD. Transcranial stab wounds: morbidity and medicolegal awareness. *Surg Neurol.* 1991;35:294–299.
295. Ström C. Injuries due to violent crimes. *Med Sci Law.* 1992;32:123–132.
296. Dannenberg AL, Parver LM, Fowler CJ. Penetrating eye injuries, related to assault. *Arch Ophthalmol.* 1992;110:849–852.
297. Kitahara T, Okada K, Takagi H, Ohwada T, Yada K. Transorbital penetrating brain injuries. Report of six cases. *Proceedings of the 4th conference of the Japanese Society of Neurotraumatology.* 1981;87–93.
298. Kosaki H, Nakamura N, Toriyama Y. Penetrating injuries to the oropharynx. *J Laryngol Otol.* 1992;106:813–816.
299. Pitner SE. Carotid thrombosis due to intraoral trauma. *N Engl J Med.* 1966;274:764–767.
300. Bickerstaff ER. Aetiology of acute hemiplegia in childhood. *Br Med J.* 1964;2: 82–87.
301. Dooling JA, Bell WE, Whitehurst WR. Penetrating skull wound from a pair of scissors: Case report. *J Neurosurg.* 1976;26:636–638.
302. Franklin GC. Death from puncture of the brain by a crochet-hook. *Lancet.* 1876;1:667.
303. Sykes PJ. An unusual penetrating injury of the cheek. A case report. *Injury.* 1973;4:347–349.
304. Markham JW, McCleve DE, Lynge HN. Penetrating cranio-cerebral injuries. *Neurosurgery.* 1964;21:1095–1097.
305. Hengerer AS, De Groot TR, Rivers RJ, Pettee DS. Internal carotid artery thrombosis following soft palate injury. A case report and review of 16 cases. *Laryngoscope.* 1984;94:1571–1574.
306. Smyth DA, Fenton J, Timon C, McShane DP. Occult pharyngeal perforation secondary to 'pencil injuries'. *J Laryngol Otol.* 1996;110:901–903.
307. Key SN, McCrummen TD. Foreign body in the brain. *JAMA.* 1932;99:1502.

308. Kenigsberg K, Ashley R, DiCarmine F. Unusual injury caused by a pencil. *J Pediatr Surg.* 1995;30:891–892.
309. Bowen DI. Self-inflicted orbito-cranial injury with a plastic ball-point pen. *Br J Ophthalmol.* 1971;55:427–430.
310. Sarvesvaran ER. Fatal penetrating orbital injuries. *Med Sci Law.* 1991;31: 261–263.
311. Betz P, Wilske J, Penning R. Perforationsverletzungen des Orbitadachs durch Regenschirmspitze. *Ophthalmologe.* 1994;91:46–48.
312. Hewitt F. Perforation of the roof of the orbit by a lead pencil with injury to the brain. *Trans Pathol Soc London.* 1847–1848;1:188–189.
313. Akgüner M, Atabey A, Top H. A case of self-inflicted intraorbital injury: wooden foreign body introduced into the ethmoidal sinus. *Ann Plast Surg.* 1998;41:422–424.
314. Stern WE. Penetration of the intracranial cavity by an object driven through the orbit. *Surg Neurol.* 1994;41:83.
315. Teeuw van. Balpen in het oor; automutulatie bij een psychotische patient. *Ned Tijdschr Geneeskunde.* 1997;141:864.
316. Jackson JH. Fracture of orbital plate of frontal bone and perforation into lateral ventricle of the brain. *Lancet.* 1884;1:205.
317. Wronski J, Tota J. [Cerebral complications following injury to the orbit with a pencil.] English abstract. *Neurol Neurochir Policy.* 1971;5:597–600.
318. Anonymous. Wound of orbit by a tobacco-pipe. *Lancet.* 1831–1832;1: 715–716.
319. Selwyn C. Deep penetration of the brain by a knife; recovery. *Lancet.* 1838;2:16.
320. Bower ED. Penetrating wound of orbit. *Br Med J.* 1879;1:547.
321. Donkin H. Left hemiplegia and left-sided deafness after wound of the brain through right orbit. *Brain.* 1882;5:554–558.
322. Johnson W. Foreign bodies in the orbital cavity. *Zentrblt Prakt Augenheilkunde.* 1894;18:449–450.
323. Koster. Verwonding der orbita door een pijpesteel. *Zbl prakt Augenhk.* 1898:251.
324. Rockliffe WC, Hainworth EM. Penetrating wound of the orbit followed by traumatic meningitis; trephining; recovery. *Trans Ophthalmol Soc UK.* 1899;19:154–159.
325. Casali A. Ferita dell'orbita penetrante nella cavità cranica; e contributo alla diagnosi oftalmoscopica dell'ematoma della guaine del nervo ottica. *Annali d'Ottalm.* 1907;36:128–137.
326. v.d. Hoeve. Eine ungewöhnliche Verletzung der Nerven. *Klin Mbl Augenheilk.* 1914;53:584.
327. Anonymous. Curious injury: fracture of the skull. *Lancet.* 1832;2:190.
328. Canuyt G, Tassowatz B, Wild Ch. Méningite purulente septique a streptocoques hémolitiques d'origine orbitaire. *Ann Otolaryng Paris.* 1933;9: 1071–1074.
329. Meyer MF, Roeting JC. Orbital abscess (following foreign body of orbit) and meningitis with recovery. *Arch Ophthalmol Chicago.* 1935;13:445–446.
330. Kuntzman J. Perforation du plafond de l'orbite par une crayon d'ardoise et méningite consecutive. *Strasbourg Med.* 1938;98:154.

331. Friermann W. Die Prognose der Gleichzeitigen Augen und Gehirnverletzungen. *Klin Mbl Augenheilk* 1941;107:265–271.
332. Kumano S. Gehirnverletzung durch die Orbita mit tödlichem Ausgang. *J Med Assoc Formosa.* 1941;40:464–469.
333. Thomas M. Knife injury. *Am J Ophthalmol.* 1942;25:210.
334. Rees TR. Perforating wound of the orbit. *Med Ann Distr Colum.* 1947;16: 548–549.
335. Lehmann. Forkenstichverletzung bei einem 14järigem Jungen in die Fissura orbitalis superior. *Dtsch Ges Wesen.* 1961;10:454.
336. Lalla M, Pillai S. Unusual penetrating injury of orbit. *Br Ophthalmol.* 1965;49:54.
337. Bochetti G, Belland F. Localizione endocrania di un grosso corpo estrano penetrato nell'orbita. *Minerva Oftalmol.* 1970;12:44–46.
338. Di Maio VJM, Di Maio DJ. An unsuspected stabwound of the brain, a case report. *Milit Med.* 1972;137:434–453.
339. Siedschlag WD, Feldman H. Zur Behandlung von transorbitalen Hirnverletzungen durch Fremdkörpereinwirkung. *Zbl Neurochir.* 1973;34:95–98.
340. Gralek M, Mert B. Cerebral complications following orbital injury caused by a branch. *Klin Oczna.* 1975;45:253–262.
341. Healy JF. Computed tomography of orbital trauma. *J Comput Tomogr.* 1982;6:1–10.
342. Krüger CJ, Seifert V, Becker H, Friedrich H, Brewitt H. Aussergewöhnliche Pfählungsverletzung von Orbita und Gehirn. *Fortschr Ophthalmol.* 1984;81: 214–216.
343. Kirkby GR. Penetrating orbitocranial injury with a snooker cue. *Br Med J.* 1986;293:1646.
344. Ravelli V, Forli C, Parenti G. Unusual penetrating craniocerebral injuries. *J Neurosurg Sci.* 1987;31:153–156.
345. Kadota K, Asakura T, Tamura M *et al.* [Transorbital intracranial penetration by chopstick. Case report]. English summary. *Neurol Med Chir Tokyo.* 1988;28: 1128–1132.
346. Sato M, Maeno K, Kawakami M, Sasaki T, Kodama N, Yago K. [A transorbital intracranial foreign body in an infant.] A report of three cases. English abstract. *Jpn J Neurosurg.* 1994;3:329–334.
347. Takakuwa T, Hakozaki S, Hurukawa K, Nakae H, Endo S. [Penetrating craniocerebral injuries during downhill skiing.] English abstract. *Neurol Surg.* 1994;22:477–479.
348. Potapov AA, Eropkin SV, Kornienko VN *et al.* Late diagnosis and removal of a large wooden foreign body in the cranio-orbital region. *J Craniofac Surg.* 1996;7:311–314.

Additional literature

Freiwald MJ. Penetrating injuries of the orbit [editorial]. *Milit Med.* 1979; 144:47.

Schönbauer HR. Tintenstiftverletzungen. *Klin Med Osterr Z Wiss Prakt Med.* 1966;21:453–454.

Brock L, Tanenbaum HL. Retention of wooden foreign bodies in the orbit. *Can J Ophthalmol.* 1980;15:70–72.

Hamilton JG. Orbital injury and carotico-cavernous fistulae. *J Neurol Neurosurg Psychiatr.* 1966;29:476.
Sebag J. Intraorbital wood [letter, comment]. *Ophthalmology.* 1990;97:1400.
Gurdjian ES, Gurdjian ES. Acute head injuries. *Surg Gynecol Obstet.* 1978;146:805–820.
Eber CT. Foreign body in both orbits. *Am J Ophthalmol.* 1940;23:318–320.
Natori Y, Rhoton AL Jr. Microsurgical anatomy of the superior orbital fissure. *Neurosurgery.* 1955;36:762–775.
Van der Straeten M. Traumatisme de l'orbite par pénétration de la pointe d'une parapluie. *Soc Belge Ophthalmol.* 1911;14:37–38.
Kosven AM. [On the surgical treatment of penetrating orbito-cranio-cerebral wounds.] *Vopr Neirohir.* 1976;31:47–48.
Granicki A, Kopera M, Majchrzak H. [Removal of a foreign body penetrating through the orbit into the cranial cavity.] English abstract. *Neurol Neurochir Pol Suppl.* 1992;1:353–355.
Sadar ES, Jane JA, Lewis LW, Adelman LS. Traumatic aneurysms of the intracranial circulation. *Surg Gynaecol Obstet.* 1973;137:59–67.

Not available:

Ferguson FN. A penetrating wound of the skull and brain. *NY Med J.* 1896;64:360.
Calmettes L, Deodati F, Bec. *Rev Oto-Neurol.* 1954;20:377–378.
Eckerlein E. *Inaugural Dissertation,* Köningsberg, 1887.
Evatt EW. Ice-pick through orbit: case report. *J S Carolina Med J.* 1947;43:236.
France. *Guy's Hosp Rep.* 1855; series III, vi: p. 58.
Ferguson FN. A penetrating wound of the skull and brain. *NY Med J.* 1896;64:300.
Fowler EP. Penetrating wound through the orbit into the middle fossa. *Arch Ophthalmol.* 1927;10:190.(?)
Pechin, Deschamps. Traumatisme orbitaire et hemiplegie alternante consecutive. *Bull Soc Opht Paris.* 1908;10:3.
Pepper W. Punctured wound of orbit. *Am J Med Sci.* 1886;52:427.
Perumainer M. Paraorbital, orbital and ocular injuries seen in a forensic department. *Trans OS Ceylon.* 1976;25:19–20.
Samelsohn. Griffelverletzung der Orbita mit nachvolgendem Abszess des Stirnhirns. *Dtsch Med Wochenschr.* 1894;20 Sept.
Zirm. Stichverletzung des Orbitaldaches mit letalen Ausgang. *Zentrallbl f prackt Augenheilk.* 1901;15:87.

List of reprints of illustrations from other authors

CHAPTER 1

Figure 1: Kahler RJ, Tomlinson FH, Eisen DP, Masel JP. Orbitocranial penetration by a fern: case report. *Neurosurgery*. 1998;42:1370–1373. [25] p. 1370. With permission of Dr Kahler and the Publisher, Lippincott, Williams and Wilkins.

Figure 2: Wertheim S. Zur Kasuistik der durch die Orbita erfolgten Fremdkörperverletzungen des Gehirns. *Inaugural Dissertation*, Giessen, 1904. [19] Title page.

Figure 3: Coqueret MP. Contribution à l'etude des plaies pénétrantes du crane par la voie orbitaire. In: Steinheil G, ed. *Thèse de Paris*, Paris. 1905. [20] Title page.

CHAPTER 2

Figure 6: Picture from *Bijbelse vertellingen voor onze kleintjes* by W.G. van der Hulst pictured by J.H. Isings, bldz. 103, 18e druk, publisher J.J. Groen en Zoon, 1994, Leiden, with permission from D.L. Aangeenburg.

Figure 7: Picture: *The deathbed of Henry 2*. From *Neurosurgery*, vol. 41, no. 6. blz. 1452 (Dec '97). With permission from the Publisher, Lippincott, Williams and Wilkins.

CHAPTER 4

Figures 8 and 9: Martial R. De l'hemiplégie traumatique. *Nouv Icon Salpêtr.* 1900;8:209–242. [63] pp. 383 and 387.

CHAPTER 5

Figure 10: Lasky JB, Epley D, Karesch JW. Household objects as a cause of self-inflicted orbital apex syndrome. *J Trauma*. 1997;42:555–558. [103] Figure 4. With permission from Dr J.W. Karesch and the Publisher, Lippincott, Williams and Wilkins.

CHAPTER 7

Figures 17, 18 and 23b: Weisman RA. Surgical anatomy of the orbit. *Otolaryngol Clin N Am.* 1988; 21:1–12. [125] Figures 1, 2 and 7, pp. 2, 4 and 9. Permission granted by the Publisher, W.B. Saunders Company (Julie Lawley).

Figure 19: Asbury CC, Castillo M, Mukherji SK. Review of computed tomographic imaging in acute orbital trauma. *Emerg Radiol.* 1995;2:367–375. [126] p. 368, Figure 1a,b,c. With permission from Dr M. Castillo and the Editor-in-Chief, Dr T.E. Keats.

Figure 23a: Dogliotti AM. Technique et indications de la ventriculographie cérébrale par la voie transvoûte-orbitaire. *Bull Memb Soc Natl Chir.* 1934;Seance II, Tome LX, no. 25. [13] p. 1019.

CHAPTER 8

Figure 26: De Villiers JC. Stab wounds of brain and skull. In: Vinken OJ, Bruyn JW, eds. *Handbook of Clinical Neurology,* Vol 1. Amsterdam: North Holland Publ. Co. 1975:477–503. [2] Figure 21. Title out of print; rights reverted to the author; author's address unknown.

Figure 27: Zentner J, Hassler W, Petersen D. A wooden foreign body penetrating the superior orbital fissure. *Neurochirurgia.* 1991;34:188–190. [157] p. 189, Figure 3. Permission granted by the Publisher, Georg Thieme Verlag Stuttgart.

CHAPTER 9

Figure 28: Anderson RL, Carroll TF, Harvey JT, Myers MG. Petriellidum (allescheria) boydii orbital and brain abscess treated with intravenous miconazole. *Am J Ophthalmol.* 1984;97:771–775. [93] p. 771, Figure 1. With permission from Elsevier Science.

CHAPTER 10

Figure 29: Mono J, Hollenberg RD, Harvey JT. Occult transorbital intracranial penetrating injuries. *Ann Emerg Med.* 1986;15:589–591. [75] Figures 1, 2 and 3. Reproduced with kind permission from Dr John Harvey and the Publisher, Mosby Inc., St Louis, MO, USA (Chidi Ukabam, Illustrations and Permissions Coordinator, 4.5.99).

CHAPTER 11

Figure 30: Bank DE, Carolan PL. Cerebral abscess formation following ocular trauma: A hazard associated with common wooden toys. *Pediatr Emerg Care.*

1993;9:285–288. [90] p. 286, Figure 1. Reproduced in this book with kind permission from Tobias Wechsler, Permissions Editor, Lippincott, Williams and Wilkins.

CHAPTER 14

Figure 31: Hsu CHY, Wang SJ. CSF leakage into the orbit demonstrated by Tc-99m DTPA cisternography. *Clin Nucl Med.* 1994;19:463. [291] Figure 2. Reproduced here with kind permission from Tobias Wechsler, Permissions Editor, Lippincott, Williams and Wilkins.

CHAPTER 15

Figure 35: Kitahara T, Okada K, Takagi H, Ohwada T, Yada K. Transorbital penetrating brain injuries. Report of six cases. *Proceedings of the 4th conference of the Japanese Society of Neurotraumatology.* 1981;87–93. p. 90, [297] Figure 5. With kind permission from Dr. Takao Kitahara. Kitasato University, Sagamihara, Japan.

CHAPTER 17

Figure 39a: Ildan F, Bagdatoglu H, Boyar B, Doganay M, Cetinalp E, Karadayi A. The nonsurgical treatment of penetrating orbito-cranial injury. *J Trauma.* 1994;36:116–118. [261] p. 116, Figures 1 and 2 (same case as Figure 39b). Reproduced in this book with kind permission of the Publisher, Lippincott, Williams and Wilkins.

Figure 39b: Oguz M, Aksungur EH, Atilla E, Altay M, Soyupak SK, Ildan F. Orbitocranial penetration of a pencil: extraction under CT control. *Eur J Radiol.* 1993;17:85–87. [160] p. 86, Figure 1. Reprinted with permission from Elsevier Science.

CHAPTER 19

Figure 45: Hewitt F. Perforation of the roof of the orbit by a lead pencil with injury to the brain. *Trans Pathol Soc London.* 1847–1848;1:188–189. [312] Title page.

CHAPTER 20

Figure 46: Albert DM, Burns WP, Scheie HG. Severe orbitocranial foreign-body injury. *Am J Ophthalmol.* 1965;60:1109. [161] p. 1109, Figures 1 and 5. Reprinted with kind permission from Elsevier Science.

Figure 47: Greene KA, Dickman CA, Smith KA, Kinder EJ, Zabramski JM. Self-inflicted orbital and intracranial injury with a retained foreign body. *Surg Neurol.* 1993;40:499–503. [264] p. 500, Figure 1a,b,c. Reprinted with kind permission from Elsevier Science.

Figure 48: Lasky JB, Epley D, Karesch JW. Household objects as a cause of self-inflicted orbital apex syndrome. *J Trauma.* 1997;42:555–558. [103] Figures 1 and 2. Reproduced here by courtesy of Dr J.W. Karesch and the Publisher, Lippincott, Williams and Wilkins.

INDEX

abducens nerve, injury 85–6
accident 94–5
  age, distribution 94(fig.)
  gender 94(fig.)
  objects used 95(fig.)
aggression 25–6, 91–3
  gender 91(fig.)
  objects used 91(fig.)
air, intracranial 1(fig.)
ala major, perforation 47
alcohol 52
amaurosis, post-traumatic 84
anatomical data 27–38
angiography 20, 69–70, 87
  carotid artery thrombosis 74
  subarachnoid hemorrhage 60
  traumatic aneurysm 71
anterior choroidal artery 88
anterior cranial fossa 10–11, 27
anterior orbital opening 12
antibiotic therapy 78–9
aphasia 17
arachnoid space 36(fig.)
auto-enucleation 108

Bacillus licheniformis 78
ballpoint pen injuries 105–7, 109(fig.)
  suicide attempt 111–12
blindness
  acute 84
  injuries by umbrellas 113
  suicide attempt 112
blink reflex 40
bone fragments 42
brain 1
  cadavers, tests 15
brain abscess 11, 80, 82
  surgical treatment 77
brainstem 44–5
  penetration 50
Broca region 15
bullet wound 10–11

cadavers, experimental research 15–19
canalis opticus 1, 43
  orbital wall, location of penetration 42(table)
  perforation through 45–6
carotid artery 35
  compression 74
  injury 36(fig.), 86–90
    angiography 74
  internal 18–19
  thrombosis 74
    occlusion through 80
  traumatic aneurysm 54
carotid cavernous fistula 11, 61, 80
  treatment, embolization 34
caudate nucleus 17
cavernous sinus 19
central retinal artery 84
cerebello-pontine angle 46
cerebellum 17, 19
cerebral complications 80–4
cerebral symptoms 23, 49
cerebrospinal fluid (CSF)
  blood finding 54
  cyst 86
  fistula 52, 74, 80
    closure 77
  leakage 43, 53, 83
    orbit 87(fig.)
chemosis 53
chiasma 16(fig.), 17
children 23–5, 38–9
civilian injuries 11

clinical presentation 48–50
clivus 19
Clostridium perfringens 78
complications 80–90
  intracranial 2
computerized tomography
    (CT) 59–66
  foreign bodies 61–6
concept, definition 12–14
conjunctiva 41
  injury 53
contralateral injury 46
contralateral mammilary tubercle 17
Coqueret's thesis 3, 5(fig.), 10
corne sphenoidale 17
corpus striatum 17
"coupe de pédonclé" 16(fig.)
cranio-orbital penetrating injury,
    reverse penetration 41
craniotomy
  indications 71–2
  open-and-see method 72–3, 75
  pull-and-observe method 73–5
  wait-and-see method 75
cuneus 17
cysternography
  metrizamide 86
  Tc-99m DTPA 87(fig.)

De Sedibus et Causis Morborum 7
diabetes insipidus 43, 46
diagnosis 49
dura 11, 13, 42
  healing tendency 32

ecchymosis 53
echography 57
empyema, subdural 9
epidural hematoma 84
epilepsy 11, 80
ethmoid bone 19, 29(fig.), 30, 40
ethmoid cribrosa 77
ethmoid sinus 27, 28(fig.)
ethmoidal air cells 28(fig.), 30
evaluation, initial 48–50
examination, physical 51–6
  history 51–2
  neurological 54–6
  ophthalmologic 52–4
exophthalmos, pulsating 85–6, 89
extraocular muscles 39
eye pulsations 85
eye socket 27, 29
eyeball 11, 39
  anatomy 34
  examination 53
  high/low-velocity injury 13
eyelid
  injury, second reflex 10
  lower 41
    cadaver, tests 15
    wound 1(fig.)
  upper 41

facio-orbital injury 13
fall injuries 93(fig.), 96–102
  age, distribution 98(figs)
  children 97
  considerations, pathogenic 100–2
  gender 99(fig.)
  mortality 101
  objects used 99(fig.)
  pencil injury 96–7
fall trauma 4, 25, 26(table), 42
foreign bodies
  radio-opaque 58
  removal 52
    hemorrhage, fatal 52
  wood
    magnetic resonance
      imaging 64–6
    ultrasonography 57–8
fossa pterygo-palatina 38
frontal leucotomy, psychiatric
    patients 33–4
frontal lobe 1, 43
frontal nerve 35(fig.)
frontal sinus 27, 28(fig.)
fundus
  examination 53
  pale edematous 84

Glasgow Coma Scale 54, 61
glucose oxidative paper tests 53
grey matter 17

hemiplegia 54
historical aspects 7–11
homolateral peduncle 16(fig.), 17
horizontal gaze paresis 54
hydrocephalus 85–6
hypo-dysesthesis 50
hypothalamus 31, 43, 104
  penetration 50

incidence 23–26
  age 25–6
  gender 24–6
  right/left orbit 24
infection 80–3
infraorbital nerve 30, 31(fig.)
infratemporal fossa 38
interior orbital fissure 29, 38, 42(table)
internal capsule 17, 54
interval, symptom-free 56–7
intracerebral hematoma 46, 74, 116
intraventricular hemorrhage 8

kinetic energy 13, 100

lacrimal nerve 35(fig.)
lamina cribrosa 1, 27, 30, 42(table), 46–7, 77
lamina papyracea 30, 43, 46
Lancet (1886, 1897), histories 9
levator palpebrae superioris 35(fig.)
literature, reviews of patients 118–37
  list (1818–1999) 124–37
lumbar puncture, air insufflation 54

magnetic resonance imaging (MRI) 66–9
  foreign bodies, wood 64–6
mammilary body 16(fig.)
Marcus-Gunn pupil 84
maxilla 29(fig.)
maxillary sinus 27, 28(fig.)
medial canthus 17, 46
  cadaver, tests 36
medicolegal aspects 116–17
medulla oblongata 15
meningitis 7, 9–10, 43, 82, 89
  mortality 11
  recurrent 52, 80
middle cerebral artery 18
morbidity 113–15
mortality 113–15
"movement de recul instinctif" 10, 42

nasociliary nerve 35(fig.)
neck stiffness 50
neuroimaging 57–70
neurosurgeon, examination 2
nucleus amygdaloideus 19

Observationes de affectibus capitis 7
occipital bone 15
ocular nerve, injury 50
oculomotor nerve 15
  injury 85–6
olfactorius nerve 32
ophthalmic artery 35(fig.), 84–5
ophthalmologist, examination 2
ophthalmoplegia 55(fig.)
optic foramen 19
optic nerve 31(fig.), 35(fig.), 53
  damage 84–5
  lesion 11
optical canal 10, 13, 27–8, 36–7
  "dead body" tests 15
optical tract 17–19
orbit 1, 20
  anatomy 27
  anterior opening, penetration 40
  radiographs 58–9
  stab wounds 19
orbital complications 84–6
orbital floor 17
  anatomy 29–30
  penetration, location 42(table)
  perforation 46–7
orbital injury, penetrating 12–13
orbital lesion, blunt 13
orbital roof 7, 10–11, 15, 19
  anatomy 29–30
  children 30, 58
  CT imaging 31(fig.)
  displaced fracture 60(fig.)

orbital roof (continued)
inside 33(fig.)
outside 32(figs)
penetration, location 42(table)
perforation through 42–3
os frontale 29(fig.), 40
os palatinum 29(fig.)
os zygomaticum 29(fig.), 30, 40

palsy, gaze 50
paralysis 11
flaccid, homolateral 20
pathogenesis 39–47
pencil injury 96, 97(fig.), 99, 105–7
child, fatal 102
penduncle 54
penetrating injuries, low/high-velocity 12–13
penetrating object/missile
kinetic energy 13
nature 20–2
perforating injuries 12
personality, changes 80
Petriellidium (*Allescheria*) *boydii* 78
petrosal bone 19
pneumocephalus 71, 81, 83
pneumoencephalus, tension 77
pons 19
porencephalia 84
porencephalic cysts 81
posterior cranial fossa 19, 36(fig.)
space-occupying lesion 86
prevention 116–17
proptosis 34, 53
publications, year of 4, 6(fig.)
puntura transorbituria 32–3

radiographs, conventional 58–9
regio calcarina 17
retinal ischaemia 84

sclera 39, 53
perforation 84
self-inflicted eye injury 108
sinus cavernosus 34–5, 43, 45, 54
foreign body, removal 74
injury 80, 86–90
perforation 88–90
puncture 18(fig.)
sinus maxillaris 13
sinus sphenoidalis 20, 28(fig.), 46
skull 1
base 18
zones 18
radiographs 58–9
sphenoid bone 29(fig.)
splenium 16(fig.)
stab wounds 3, 12
Staphylococcus aureus 78
striate body 15

subarachnoid hemorrhage 54, 88
angiography 60
sudden death 88
suicide 25, 26(table), 51, 108–12
superior orbital fossa 1, 10, 13, 18, 20, 27
anatomy 29(fig.), 35(fig.)
anterior orbital opening 37(fig.)
"dead body" tests 15
intracranial roots 36(fig.)
penetration 43–5
orbital wall, location 42(table)
sylvian fissure 15, 17

temporal fossa 10, 27
temporal lobe 45–6
tetanus antitoxin 54
thalamus 17
transorbital stab, structures damaged 43(fig.)
traumatic aneurysm 74, 81, 88
development 86
traumatic tap 56
treatment 71–7
trepanation 11
frontal, psychiatric patients 34
fronto-temporal 72
trigeminal nerve 102
injury 85–6
trochlear nerve 35(fig.)
injury 85–6

ultrasonography 57–8
umbrellas 10–11, 103–4
fall injury 96

left orbit injuries, compared with knife 92(fig.)
mortality after injury 91
patients, age distribution 103(fig.)

vascular complications 80, 86–90
vascular spasms 87
velocity 13
ventricle system 11
ventriculitis 82
vision prognosis 85
visually evoked potentials 85

Wagner's pioneering osteoplastic craniotomy 11
Wertheim's dissertation/thesis 3, 4(fig.), 10
wood, density values 62(table), 63
wooden objects, morbidity 21
wound cultures 54

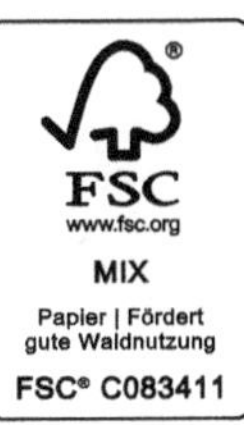

Zeitfracht Medien GmbH
Ferdinand-Jühlke-Straße 7
99095 Erfurt, Deutschland
produktsicherheit@kolibri360.de